Care of the Person with Dementia
Interprofessional practice and education

With rising life expectancies, the prevalence of dementia has increased to such an extent that it is now recognised as a National Health Priority Area. *Care of the Person with Dementia* responds to the urgent need for health practitioners to take an innovative approach to this challenge. The first Australian text of its kind, this book combines evidence-based resources with interprofessional education and practice. It explores the ethical, social and environmental repercussions of dementia to provide a comprehensive overview of dementia care in an Australian context.

Care of the Person with Dementia is structured around a model of interprofessional education and practice (IPE) tailored to dementia care. This model incorporates the context of care, an important element missing from other recognised models of IPE. Throughout the book, the principles of IPE are explained within the context of dementia, drawing on exemplars from a body of current, well-researched and evaluated dementia practice.

Written by experienced academics, and providing national and international perspectives, this is a unique and crucial resource for students, health educators and health professionals wanting to develop collaborative skills and professional knowledge in the management of dementia.

Dawn Forman is Visiting Professor of Interprofessional Education at the University of Derby, and Adjunct Professor at Curtin University.

Dimity Pond is Professor of General Practice at the University of Newcastle.

Care of the Person with Dementia

Interprofessional practice and education

Edited by

Dawn Forman and Dimity Pond

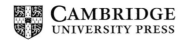
CAMBRIDGE
UNIVERSITY PRESS

CAMBRIDGE
UNIVERSITY PRESS

477 Williamstown Road, Port Melbourne, VIC 3207, Australia

Cambridge University Press is part of the University of Cambridge.

It furthers the University's mission by disseminating knowledge in the pursuit of education, learning and research at the highest international levels of excellence.

www.cambridge.org
Information on this title: www.cambridge.org/9781107678453

© Cambridge University Press 2015

First published 2015

Cover designed by Tanya De Silva-McKay
Typeset by Aptara Corp.
Printed in Singapore by Markono Print Media Pte Ltd

A catalogue record for this publication is available from the British Library

A Cataloguing-in-Publication entry is available from the catalogue of the National Library of Australia at www.nla.gov.au

ISBN 978-1-107-67845-3 Paperback

Foreword

Over the past decade there has been a significant movement towards interprofessional practice (IPP) and education within health care, as a key strategy to increase the effectiveness of health care delivery. Recent studies and systematic reviews have shown that IPP is well received by clinicians, can change their perceptions and attitudes, and is related to improvements in knowledge, skills and collaborative practice. There is a growing body of research showing the positive impact of IPP approaches on healthcare processes, patient satisfaction and clinical outcomes.

For people living with dementia and their carers, there will be many critical points across the trajectory of disease when they will seek – or be offered – advice, treatment, care and support. The organisation, delivery and quality of the health care they receive, and the important relationships that are formed in the process, can make the difference between a seamless healthcare journey that enhances overall quality of daily life or a fragmented, stressful series of encounters that makes the journey more difficult. Recent international and Australian initiatives in interprofessional dementia care have illustrated the potential benefits of this type of approach to the complex range of needs and issues that occur for people living with dementia and their carers.

This book is a response to the learning needs of healthcare professionals who are engaged with people living with dementia and those who care for and support them. Across 10 chapters the reader is introduced to core concepts in interprofessional dementia education and practice, interprofessional dementia care leadership, the journey of dementia, predominant philosophies of care, the evidence base in dementia care, international perspectives, collaborative skill development, ethical issues in dementia care and the intersection of interprofessional practice and care environments. The authors are predominantly Australian, come from many different disciplines, have strong histories of involvement in dementia education, treatment and care and are committed to making a difference to the healthcare experiences and daily lives of people living with dementia and their carers. The book is strengthened with input from realistic scenarios discussed through an interprofessional lens.

For any person interested in developing a greater understanding of the interprofessional approach to dementia care and support put forward by the author team, this book is a comprehensive, easy introduction. For those involved in educating and training for dementia care and support it offers a model for organising content and learning experiences and can be used alongside other theories and models. The examples used in the book to help readers think about their practice are helpful and realistic.

I confidently recommend it as a useful adjunct to dementia education and commend the authors on bringing it to the community of people dedicated to improving the daily lives of people living with dementia and their carers.

Elizabeth Beattie

Professor, Aged and Dementia Care

Director, Dementia Collaborative Research Centre: Carers and Consumers

Director, Queensland Dementia Training Study Centre School of Nursing,

Queensland University of Technology

Brisbane, 28 April 2015.

Contents

List of figures and tables

Contributors

Michael Annear is a gerontologist and research fellow in translational health services at the Wicking Dementia Research and Education Centre, Faculty of Health, University of Tasmania. Dr Annear also lectures within the Bachelor of Dementia Care and is a contributor to the international Understanding Dementia Massive Open Online Course.

Jade Cartwright (BSc Human Communication Science (First Class Hons), PhD) is a speech pathologist and lecturer at the University of Melbourne. Jade is also an adjunct lecturer at Curtin University. Jade's clinical, research and teaching interests include the psychosocial impact of communication disorders associated with dementia, including primary progressive aphasia, and the development and evaluation of novel speech pathology interventions for individuals living with dementia and their families. Jade is a strong advocate for interprofessional approaches to dementia care, and the establishment of high quality clinical placements in dementia and aged care settings to effectively train a future health workforce.

Richard Fleming (BTech (Hons), Dip Clin Psy, PhD) is a professorial fellow and Director of the New South Wales and Australian Capital Territory Dementia Training Study Centre at the University of Wollongong. Richard is a psychologist, and was the Regional Coordinator of Mental Health Services in the SE Region of New South Wales for six years, and Director of the Hammond Care Dementia Services Development Centre for 16 years. He has provided consultancy services on the care of elderly people, particularly those with dementia, in Japan, Singapore, Hong Kong, India, Canada, Norway, the UK and across Australia.

Dawn Forman (PhD, MBA, PG Dip Research, PG Dip Executive Coaching, TDCR MDCR) is Visiting Professor at the University of Derby (UK) and the University of Chichester (UK), and Adjunct Professor at Auckland University of Technology (New Zealand) and Curtin University (Australia). Dawn was a Dean of Faculty for Education Health and Science disciplines for 13 years, and over the last seven years she has worked as a consultant with universities and health services internationally. She is an associate for the Higher Education Academy and the Leadership Foundation for Higher Education, and a senior associate of Ranmore Consulting.

Heather Freegard (MSocSc (Human Services), BAppSc (OT), Churchill Fellow) was, until her recent retirement, the Project Coordinator with the WA Dementia Training Study Centre (WA DTSC), based at Curtin University. WA DTSC is one of five federally funded centres across Australia as part of the Australian government's Dementia Initiative to increase the knowledge and skills base of health professionals who are, or seeking to be, qualified at a tertiary level across primary, residential, acute and community care sectors, and working with people with dementia. The DTSCs are primarily involved in dementia-specific education and knowledge transfer for the health and aged care sector. Heather's clinical and academic career focused on the areas of gerontology and ethics, especially how people with dementia and their families are affected by health policy and the delivery of human services.

Sue Fyfe has held senior leadership and management roles at Curtin University as inaugural Dean of Teaching and Learning in the Faculty of Health Sciences, Head of School of Public Health and Professor of Medical Education for the proposed School of Medicine. She is Deputy Chair of the WA Peel Development Commission, a board member of the Maureen

Bickley Centre for Women in Leadership and member of the Perth South Coastal Medicare Local Advisory Committee. She is an epidemiologist, anatomist, speech pathologist and teacher.

Kreshnik Hoti (BPharm, MPS, AACPA, PhD) is a lecturer in the School of Pharmacy at Curtin University. He has practised both community and consultancy pharmacy. Kreshnik completed his PhD thesis on pharmacist prescribing and medication supply models to residential aged care facilities.

Jeffery Hughes (BPharm, PostGradDipPharm, MPharm, PhD, MPS, AACPA) is the former Head of the School of Pharmacy, Curtin University. He is an accredited pharmacist and part-owner of a community pharmacy. He serves on the boards of the Pharmaceutical Society of Western Australia and the Pharmaceutical Society of Australia. Jeff has received a number of state and national awards for his contribution to pharmacy education, practice and research, including the Pharmaceutical Society of Australia's Pharmacist of the Year Award in 2004, the Eric Kirk Memorial Award in 2008, the AACP Pfizer Consultant Pharmacist Award in 2009 and, most recently, the Australasian Pharmaceutical Sciences Association Medal in 2014.

Janet McCray (PhD, MSc, BSc, CertEd, RNLD, RNT) is a professor in the Department of Childhood, Social Work and Social Care at the University of Chichester in the UK. Janet is a qualitative researcher with expertise and interest in collaborative integrated care practice. She works with external agencies in the public and private sector to develop the health and social care workforce through building positive approaches in leadership and management.

Stephan Millett (BEcon, BA(Hons), PhD) is a professor of philosophy specialising in ethics, attached to the School of Occupational Therapy and Social Work at Curtin. He was formerly Chair of the Human Research Ethics Committee at Curtin University. He is a former journalist and newspaper editor who taught journalism at Curtin University for 12 years.

Lyn Phillipson (BAppSc, MPH, PhD) is a senior lecturer in the School of Health and Society at the University of Wollongong. She was responsible for the development of a Knowledge Translation (KT) Framework for use within the National Dementia Training and Study Centres in Australia (2011–13) and is currently involved in the development of an evaluation tool to assess their KT outcomes. Prior to her academic career, she worked as a physiotherapist in aged care and rehabilitation and as a health education officer.

Dimity Pond (MBBS, FRACGP, PhD) is Professor and Head of the Discipline of General Practice at the University of Newcastle. She is a GP with a background in high school and university teaching, and with teaching qualifications. She was part of a research team that developed Australian GP Dementia Guidelines. Professor Pond was chief investigator (CIA) on an NHMRC-funded randomised control trial of an educational intervention for dementia in general practice. She runs the primary care section of the Dementia Collaborative Research Centre and is also part of the Cognitive Decline Partnership Centre.

Acknowledgements

It is estimated that the number of Australians with dementia will reach 400 000 by 2020. So, if we do not have dementia ourselves, we will have cared for someone with dementia, either as a family member or as a health care worker. How we as a population cope with this impact needs careful consideration and planning.

The authors of this book were passionate about the need to address this issue when they started writing, and are all the more passionate as this book is completed.

The authors' resolve to make a difference is in no small part due to their personal experiences during the course of writing. Heather Freegard, along with Dawn Forman, created the vision for this book and designed the Model of Interprofessional Practice and Education – Dementia (MIPPE-D). Sadly Heather herself started with cognitive difficulties and, whilst her contributions to the book have been included, she was not able to continue with authoring the full book. In addition, Dawn's mother, Iris Forman, who had been diagnosed with dementia at the start of the book, died on 8 November 2014.

As a professor of general practice, Dimity Pond addresses the needs of individuals with dementia and their families on a daily basis. She feels equally passionate about the interprofessional team learning and working together in addressing these needs. Dimity was therefore able to smoothly step in as Heather withdrew from authoring this book.

Dawn and Dimity are very grateful for the inspiration and courage of both Heather and Iris, and to everyone who has contributed in making this book possible. They would also like to thank Jeanne Clark, for her patient editing and administrative assistance, Nina Sharpe, for all her guidance through the publishing process and Lisa Fraley, for her patience through the editing process.

Introduction to dementia

Heather Freegard, Dimity Pond and Dawn Forman

Learning outcomes

1 Describe what dementia is in broad descriptive medical terms.

2 Describe the impact of dementia on the Australian population in terms of disability burden.

3 Identify some of the key challenges for individuals and their families and carers throughout the course of the disease.

4 Reflect on the impact of culture and membership of different special needs groups on the experience of dementia.

5 Outline how interprofessional ways of working are needed in the care of people with dementia.

Key terms

- aged care services
- autonomy
- communication
- culture
- dementia
- interprofessional
- neurocognitive disorder (NCD)
- respect

Introduction

Dementia is a life limiting condition. The needs of people living with dementia are at the forefront of the minds of people concerned with receiving, resourcing, managing, providing and evaluating services for older people. In particular, there is an urgent need for

> **Dementia**
> Dementia is now referred to as a neurocognitive disorder (NCD) (American Psychiatric Association, 2013), that is, the result of chronic or progressive damage to the brain.

1

health care teams and service providers to respond in innovative ways (Productivity Commission, 2011) to address the 'mismatch of professional competencies to patient and population priorities' and the chronic shortfall in health workforces (Frenk et al., 2010; Health Workforce Australia, 2012).

As people live longer, the shape of society has changed and is continuing to change; creating both benefits and challenges that humanity has not met before. One of these challenges is the increased prevalence of dementia (Productivity Commission, 2011). Dementia embodies our greatest fears: a living death; cognitive decline; lost abilities; increasing dependence; loss of the person as others know them. While acknowledging that a person with dementia and their families require complex care and support over an extended period of years, perhaps there are lessons to be learned by society about what it means to be human and the real priorities of living and dying.

Dementia in Australia

The Australian Institute of Health and Welfare (AIHW) (2012) has estimated that, in 2011, 298 000 Australians had dementia. Sixty-two per cent were women, 74% were aged 75 and over, and 70% lived in the community. Based on projections of population ageing and growth, the number of people with dementia will reach almost 400 000 by 2020 and 900 000 by 2050. However, it is not only the total number of people with the disease that causes concern because that number is, on the whole, in line with the projected growth of the total population. Dementia causes concern because it comes with an increased burden of disease and disability.

The disability-adjusted life year (DALY) is a measure of overall burden of disease and is expressed as the number of years lost due to premature death and/or ill health, disability or injury. Premature death is a social and economic loss because that person can no longer participate and contribute to society and is measured in years of life lost (YLL). When a person's participation and contribution to society is limited through disease, disability or injury, or years of life lost due to disability (YLD), there is a cost to society for their care and assistance required. For people aged 65 or more, ischaemic heart disease is the leading cause of burden of disease. Approximately 75% of the burden is caused by YLL and 25% by YLD. Dementia is the second leading cause of overall burden of disease with approximately 75% comprising YLD, thus making it the leading cause of disability burden (AIHW, 2012).

Dementia is both a chronic and terminal condition. People with dementia also have, on average, more concomitant health conditions. Therefore, people with dementia and their families rely heavily on health and **aged care services**. People who identify as Aboriginal and Torres Strait Islander, or are from culturally and linguistically diverse backgrounds, or other special needs groups, are under-represented in numbers of people who access services. Fifty-three per cent of people living with dementia reside in the community and place a substantial demand on informal carers – for example, family, friends and neighbours – some providing as much as 40 hours of care per week (AIHW, 2012).

Aged care services
The Australian government subsidises many different types of aged care services to help people stay at home. They are there to help people stay as independent as they can through a system that provides fair and equitable access to services for all older people living in Australia.

Special needs groups

Australian **culture** and lifestyles reflect great diversity. The non-health needs and preferences of some older Australians can be very different from those who live in the mainstream. Many have experienced stigma as a consequence of their identity or preferred lifestyle. The *Aged Care Act 1997* specifies that people who identify as Aboriginal and Torres Strait Islander, are culturally and linguistically diverse, are living in remote or rural communities, and are financially and socially disadvantaged have special care needs to be addressed. In addition, the Allocation Principles 1997, associated with the Act, identified veterans, the homeless and people brought up in care as also having special needs. Other groups with needs that differ in certain ways but not specifically identified in legislation include people with a disability who cannot live independently in the community; ageing people with physical and/or mental disabilities; older gay, lesbian, bisexual, transgender and intersex people; and older refugees (Productivity Commission, 2011). For each of these specifically identified groups, and any other minority group, the experience of dementia can be more complicated. Consideration of the person's cultural background, gender, race, ethnicity, religious belief, disability, social and family considerations, other medical conditions, and the availability of services all need to be taken into consideration for each individual.

Culture
The main definition of culture used in this book is: 'Culture is all aspects of life, the totality of meanings, ideas and beliefs shared by individuals within a group of people. Culture is learned, it includes language, values, norms, customs.' (http://www. design.iastate. edu/NAB/about/ thinkingskills/ cultural_context/ cultural.html).

What is a neurocognitive disorder?

Dementia, now referred to as a neurocognitive disorder (American Psychiatric Association (APA), 2013), is the result of chronic or progressive damage to the brain. It is the changed and changing behaviour and actions, such as **communication** difficulties, memory loss, mood and difficulties completing everyday tasks, that provide the external evidence for the altered brain physiology. In the beginning the changes of behaviour are often subtle and insidious in nature and easily ignored or explained away as a normal part of ageing, or a reflection of the person's personality, or a natural reaction to stress or changed circumstances. It is, therefore, virtually impossible to determine when the disease begins.

> **Communication**
> An exchange of information between individuals using speech, visual aids, body language, writing or behaviour.

Major **neurocognitive disorder (NCD)** is a syndrome, that is, a cluster of symptoms which when seen together indicate changes in the brain *but* each symptom can have many causes. It is an umbrella term to describe a collection of disease processes that cause different sequences of brain damage, and variations in appearance and severity of symptoms (APA, 2013). So not only can each sign or symptom be caused by something other than a neurocognitive deficit, for example, vision loss or lack of sleep, but the NCD can have many differing causes, for example, Lewy Body disease or Alzheimer's disease. This can make diagnosis difficult as there are currently no easily tested biomarkers to confirm a diagnosis. Rather it is generally based on elimination of other possible causes of the behavioural changes, such as delirium, depression, physical ill health or medication side effects. Brain imaging may prove helpful, if feasible (Buntinx et al., 2011; Brodaty et al., 2013).

> **Neurocognitive disorder (NCD)**
> Neurocognitive disorder is an umbrella term to describe a collection of disease processes that cause different sequences of brain damage, and variations in appearance and severity of symptoms (American Psychiatric Association, 2013).

As dementia progresses, the concomitant memory and cognitive problems, and behaviour change make it an easier diagnosis to make. However, it is important that health care teams explicitly discuss the diagnosis with families once it is clear, as what may be clear to a health professional may not be clear to the family. Many family carers report great relief at getting a diagnosis, and being able at last to understand what is happening and what is likely to happen in the future with their loved one (Phillips, Pond & Shell, 2010).

Even with the best support, the person with dementia will experience profound changes in their life as a result of the disease and present challenges for carers. Few people will not be directly affected as they, siblings, parents, grand-parents, colleagues and friends experience the disease. This raises many questions about how society can or should support people with dementia and how research into dementia and dementia care is prioritised (Nuffield Council on Bioethics, 2009). Fundamental ethical issues, such as the need to balance **autonomy** with the person's safety, are an everyday problem in the journey of dementia (Department of Health (UK), 2010).

> **Autonomy**
> The capacity to make rational, uncoerced and informed decisions about the things that affect one's life.

Dementia is a terminal illness. The terminal stages of dementia are accompanied by profound changes in cognition to the point where the person may no longer be able to name their family members or indeed communicate intelligibly with them. Ultimately dementia causes death.

Internationally, improvements in public health (water supply, sewerage, occupational health and safety), social health (housing, education, employment) and medical interventions (immunisation, surgery, pharmacology, birthing practices) enable more people to live longer, healthier lives into old age despite ongoing conflict and war between and among human groups, inequitable access to resources and the increasing instability of climate and weather. However, all humans are faced with often uncomfortable truths: we must eventually die and before we die most will experience a period of decline of physical and/or cognitive abilities.

In societies, such as those in Australia, where participation in work and social life according to ability is the norm, people with disabilities, the infirm and the aged can be invisible and lack value within a community. Death is seen as a time of final messages, instructions and farewells to the family and friends who come to pay their respects.

Death and dying remains a taboo subject in contemporary society perpetually searching for longevity, with youth, vigour and independence synonymous with beauty. The development of medicine and health care in the twentieth century, and the establishment of the modern hospital, reinforced a view of dying and death as a failure, shrouding the event from all but a few close relatives (McGann, 2013); and even then many people do not attend a funeral until adulthood. Death and dying is barely mentioned in university undergraduate courses, so that when finally let loose on the trusting public those that are relied upon for knowledge, care and support often rely on the families of the dying and the dying themselves to offer them knowledge and support.

It is important that health care teams are prepared to deal with terminal illness and are taught to work with people and their families in those enormously important terminal phases. Ethical issues here are also important. Health care teams need to be trained to recognise when medical treatment is futile, and allow people to die with dignity, preferably in a place where they are comfortable and familiar, rather than in the terrifying and unfamiliar environment of the hospital.

Increase of people living with dementia

Alzheimer's Australia's key facts and statistics (Strivens & Craig, 2014) indicate that in 2014 more than 332 000 Australians had dementia. Furthermore:

- The number of Australians with dementia is expected to increase to 400 000 in less than 10 years and to about 900 000 by 2050.
- Each week there are 1700 new cases of dementia in Australia; by 2050 this number is expected to increase to 7400.
- About 24 700 people in Australia have younger onset dementia (a diagnosis of dementia at ≤65 years, including people as young as 30 years).
- Three in 10 people >85 years, and around one in 10 people >65 years has dementia.
- About 1.2 million Australians care for someone with dementia.
- Dementia is the third leading cause of death in Australia and the third cause of disability burden overall.
- On average, symptoms of dementia are noticed by family members three years before a firm diagnosis is made.

At the same time as seeing an increase of people with dementia, we are seeing a decrease of people in the younger age groups who could choose to become health professionals. The Australian Bureau of Statistics (2014) indicates that, in 2012, people aged 65 years and over made up 14% of Australia's population. This is projected to increase to 22% in 2061 and to 25% in 2101. The proportion of people aged less than 15 years is projected to decrease from 19% in 2012 to 17% in 2061 and 16% in 2101.

It's not all doom and gloom

With all great challenges come great opportunities. Increasingly Australians are living longer and healthier lives. Dementia as a leading cause of death can be seen as a positive consequence of this success. While numbers of people living with dementia increase, and their need for supportive care increases, so too does the total population of Australia. So, with appropriate societal will, there are and will be adequate resources and employees. As each family is directly involved, their commitment and access to service provision will improve and grow. While research is still discovering more questions than answers, the pieces are beginning to indicate possible treatments that can allay some of the more distressing symptoms. As Australia's cultural diversity increases and challenges current health structures and beliefs, the differing viewpoints and experiences can broaden and strengthen our understanding of the human condition.

How things are done, so that people with dementia feel valued as individuals, is often more important than the particular structure or format of services. Families as equal partners in care, alongside the person living with dementia, the health care teams and the care workers, will produce relationships of trust based on mutual **respect** (Nuffield Council on Bioethics, 2009).

> **Respect**
> Due regard for the feelings, wishes or rights of others.

We cannot continue with business as usual. We must try something different if we are to have sustainable, high quality, responsive care for all Australians, especially people living with dementia (Health Workforce Australia, 2012).

Interprofessional care

In order to ensure that we have professionals who can work with the growing number of older people and the increase of those who will have dementia, we need to ensure that our health care teams learn to value and appreciate working with the elderly. Our undergraduates, therefore, need to learn how to communicate with this age group, how to listen to their needs and their individual perspectives on life, and how, as professionals, they can support individuals in leading as full a life as possible. As dementia will affect a large proportion of this age group but can also affect younger people, we feel that dementia, from the initial signs and symptoms through to the care needed as a person is dying, should be part of the curriculum. We are concerned that, with fewer health professionals in the future, good communication not only between health care teams but with the individual, their carers and families is crucial. Therefore we believe that health care professionals in the future should all be **interprofessional**, and that an interprofessional way of working is paramount for the care of people with dementia.

> **Interprofessional**
> The terms 'interprofessional education/practice/teamwork' etc. have been defined by various groups. These terms are often used interchangeably. Where we simply use the term 'interprofessional', we do so when two or more professions are working collaboratively together.

Conclusion

The number of people with dementia is increasing in Australia. Our current and future health care professionals must be educated to recognise the needs of these individuals at each stage of the disease. They must also to be able to communicate with each other, as well as with the person with dementia, their carers and their families. We hope that this book helps our current and future health care professionals in considering the needs of people with dementia.

Self-directed learning activities

1   What changes in the workforce are needed to meet the needs of new cases of dementia in Australia between now and 2050?
2   Can you think of any ways in which the workforce might be improved other than by an increase in numbers? Think in particular of ways in which different professionals work together.
3   How might the gap between first symptoms and diagnosis be reduced? Should it be reduced?

References

American Psychiatric Association (APA). (2013). *Diagnostic and statistical manual of mental disorders* (5th edn). Arlington, VA: APA.

Australian Bureau of Statistics. (2014). Retrieved 30 March 2015 from http://www.abs.gov.au/ausstats/abs@.nsf/Lookup/3222.0main+features32012%20%28base%29%20to%202101

Australian Government. (1997). *Australian Aged Care Act 1997*. Canberra: Australian Government.

Australian Institute of Health and Welfare (AIHW). (2012). *Dementia in Australia*. Cat. No. AGE 70. Canberra: AIHW. Retrieved 30 March from http://www.aihw.gov.au/WorkArea/DownloadAsset.aspx?id=10737422943

Brodaty, H., Connors, M., Pond, D., Cumming, A. & Creasey, H. (2013). Dementia: 14 essentials of assessment and care planning. *Medicine Today*, 14(8): 18–27.

Buntinx, F., De Lepeleire, J., Paquay, L., Iliffe, S. & Schoenmakers, B. (2011). Diagnosing dementia: No easy job. *BMC Family Practice*, 12(1): 60.

Department of Health (UK). (2010). *Nothing ventured, nothing gained: Risk guidance for people with dementia*. London: DOH.

Frenk, J., Chen, L., Bhutta, Z.A., Cohen, M.D., Crisp, N., Evans, T. ... Zurayk, H. (2010). Health professionals for a new century: Transforming education to strengthen health systems in an independent world. *Lancet, 376*: 1923–58.

Health Workforce Australia. (2012). *National common health capability resource: Shared activities and behaviours in the Australian health workforce.* Adelaide: Health Workforce Australia.

McGann, S. (2013). *The production of hospice space: Conceptualising the space of caring and dying.* Surrey: Ashgate Publishing Limited.

Nuffield Council on Bioethics. (2009). *Dementia: Ethical issues.* London: Nuffield Council on Bioethics.

Phillips, J., Pond, D. & Shell, A. (2010). *No time like the present: The importance of a timely dementia diagnosis.* Scullin, ACT: Alzheimer's Australia.

Productivity Commission. (2011). *Caring for older Australians.* Report No. 53, Final Inquiry Report. Canberra: Commonwealth of Australia.

Strivens, E. & Craig, D. (2014). Managing dementia related cognitive decline in patients and their caregivers. *Caregivers: Australian Family Physician, 43*(4): 170–4.

1 The Model of Interprofessional Practice and Education – Dementia

Dawn Forman and Heather Freegard

Learning outcomes

1 Examine the competencies and capabilities required for interprofessional practice.

2 Discuss the relevance of context for working in an interprofessional manner.

3 Explain specific capabilities required in dementia care.

4 Explain the Model of Interprofessional Practice and Education – Dementia.

Key terms

- capabilities
- competencies
- dementia
- evaluation
- interprofessional
- interprofessional education (IPE)
- personhood

Introduction

In 1978, the World Health Organization stated:

> Given that effective health care requires the services of personnel with different competencies, it is essential that trainees should have

appropriate experience of such cooperative endeavours and have the ability to work towards a common goal, to communicate and share responsibility.

As community members, students and/or practitioners, we have all worked in many team environments – for example, the workplace, sport, committees, community services, and group assignments – where people with varying skills and knowledge come together to jointly achieve a goal or provide a service. Within health settings, team practice is common where a group of professionals – for example, nurse, social worker, oncologist, pharmacist and radiographer – manage the care of a specified number of patients as a coordinated group. However, very few of these experiences can be described as **interprofessional**.

Respectful working relationships with shared decision making, shared leadership and shared learning are the hallmarks of interprofessional practice (IPP). In addition to specific professional competence, other skills are required: the ability to work collaboratively; to take responsibility for your own actions and the actions of the team as a whole; to take a leadership role or follow the lead of others depending on circumstances; and the ability to provide a consistent service while under pressure.

The care of a person with **dementia** and their families is complex. Dementia is an umbrella term to describe many different causal diseases and processes, resulting in complex challenges associated with accurate diagnosis and treatment. Dementia is a progressive and life limiting condition with an unpredictable and variable trajectory from diagnosis to death. Dementia affects cognitive functions so that decision making, memory and praxis (performance of action) abilities change over time and the person requires assistance to use their remaining abilities and support to compensate for losses. This context challenges everyone's knowledge, skills and attitudes.

This chapter will outline some of the developments that have taken place internationally, not only in interprofessional competencies, but in **competencies** for dementia care, and provide a model that seeks to combine the two sets of competencies in order to provide a person-centred interprofessional model.

Interprofessional
The terms 'interprofessional education/practice/teamwork' etc. have been defined by various groups. These terms are often used interchangeably. Where we simply use the term 'interprofessional', we do so when two or more professions are working collaboratively together.

Dementia
Dementia is now referred to as a neurocognitive disorder (NCD) (American Psychiatric Association, 2013), that is, the result of chronic or progressive damage to the brain.

Competencies
Forman, Jones & Thistlethwaite (2014) define competency as the ability to 'identify specific knowledge, skills, attitudes, values and judgements that are dynamic, developmental and evolutionary'.

Models of interprofessional education and practice

The first step to **interprofessional education (IPE)** and practice is to identify and reach agreement on the specific knowledge, skills and attitudes required. Constructing a model or framework to demonstrate the multidimensional and interconnectedness of the elements helps to explain and understand the concept; to incorporate the acquisition of skills and **capabilities** into undergraduate, postgraduate and professional development programs; and to adapt or modify systems and processes to incorporate IPP into the workplace. Models and frameworks can also be used to develop tools to review or evaluate the capabilities of students and practitioners to 'work towards a common goal, to communicate and share responsibility' (Atkinson et al., 2002).

> **Interprofessional education (IPE)**
> Interprofessional education occurs when two or more professions learn with, from and about each other to improve collaboration and the quality of care (http://www.caipe.org.uk/about-us/defining-ipe/).
>
> When students from two or more professions learn about, from and with each other to enable effective collaboration and improve health outcomes (WHO, 2010).

Assessing interprofessional capabilities

Assessment of interprofessional capabilities is complex and multidimensional. Any health care educator is aware of the need to ensure that graduates entering the profession can apply evidence-based practice knowledge and skills beyond theoretical knowledge learned at university, and implement newly acquired competencies (Higgs, Andresen & Fish, 2004). As this learning is context based in the community of practice (Dahlgren, Richardson & Sjostrom, 2004), peers, role models, mentors and supervisors can significantly influence the quality of learning (Ajjawi & Higgs, 2008; Goldenberg & Iwasiw, 1993; Johnsson & Hager, 2008). Successful adaptation relies on social learning and active participation in reflection, and feedback from reliable others to judge actions and decisions (Regehr & Eva, 2007). Self-directed learning, critical thinking, reflective practice, and adaptability and flexibility are highlighted as skills for lifelong learning (Barr, 2002; Smith & Pilling, 2007). The development of these skills in the practice environment during this critical transition time facilitates graduates' successful transition

> **Capabilities**
> Forman, Jones and Thistlethwaite (2014) define capability as 'has been used in preference to competence in one IPE framework, as it is considered by some educators to reflect more optimally the necessity that learners and professionals respond and adapt to health care and systems changes'.

to the workforce (Johnsson & Hager, 2008; Smith & Pilling, 2007). Documentation of such continuing education practice after graduation is essential to retain professional registration. The following headings may be used as a guide under which evidence could be given to demonstrate continuing practice education:

- *Client/patient/person/family/community-centred care* that is effective, efficient and culturally appropriate within available resources is the primary driving force behind IPE and IPP.
- Sound socially responsible *ethical principles and values* guide service provision. Respect for autonomy, quality of life, equity and maximising benefit, and minimising harm are key principles.
- *Collaboration and collaborative practice* is strongly emphasised. The increasingly complex world of health practice means that no one person can possibly hold all the requisite knowledge, skills and attitudes to address client needs. Collaboration is more effective than teamwork, implying mutual respect, and shared leadership and authority.
- *Communication* is the most useful and effective tool to ensure collaborative practice and effective client outcomes.
- *Professionalism* includes organisational competence, reflection and conflict resolution.
- IPP requires practitioners to *establish and maintain the evidence-based knowledge, skills and attitudes* appropriate for professional registration. This encompasses the abilities to recognise limits to scope of practice and personal expertise, to seek appropriate consultation, and refer to other professionals with the required knowledge and skills.

All attributes, with the exception of the last, are generic; that is, are required by all people involved in the health needs of an individual client or client group to create a strong, flexible context in which the delivery of effective health services can occur. Facilitating the development, and **evaluation**, of interprofessional capabilities is complex and multidimensional.

Evaluation
Appraisal or value of something.

Learning and applying these skills in the workplace is further complicated because not all health care environments practise within an interprofessional approach. Whilst it can be claimed that most health care is now delivered by teams, not all teams are inclusive or work collaboratively towards a common goal, communicate effectively and share responsibility. Students and practitioners alike often find themselves in health settings where systems and processes structure practice along hierarchical and siloed lines.

Is the context in which interprofessional education and practice occurs relevant?

Health services are provided within a variety of contexts, such as:

- geographical; for example, inner city, suburban, rural or remote communities;
- service delivery; for example, acute care, emergency department, community service, rehabilitation;
- specialty; for example, orthopaedics, oncology, mental health;
- by age; for example, paediatrics, adolescence, adult and aged care services;
- funding source; for example, state government, federal government, private for profit, not-for-profit.

Likewise, preparation for professional practice occurs in many contexts, such as at universities at undergraduate and postgraduate levels, within specific professional schools and departments, and across faculties. Within each context, or combination of contexts, IPE brings great benefits to clients and service providers alike. IPE models to date reflect the health education environment in which each was developed. Methods of evaluation and standards of achievement reflect the needs of that environment. While many of the elements within the models are universal, the interaction between elements may not be, making the transfer across different working situations difficult. Each context brings with it benefits and challenges to the process. The social and physical environment, like the air we breathe, can become so familiar that it almost becomes invisible and its influences become unnoticed unless and until something major, like toxic fumes, focuses our attention. This state of invisibility removes the potential to modify the environmental contexts as important areas of service provision and improvement.

Specific capabilities for the client with dementia

The differences within dementia care contexts must be recognised if a model of interprofessional practice and education is to make a beneficial contribution to the discussion. First, such a model must acknowledge the real-world nature of clinical practice and service delivery, in addition to the realities of educational institutions. Second, the model must address the social, emotional, medical and psychological complexities that living with dementia brings.

Dementia is a complex syndrome of cognitive, behavioural and psychological symptoms with many different, and largely not understood, causations. This complexity is evident by the varying presentations and individual variations in when and how the disease affects each person with dementia. The focus on measuring and accommodating losses in function blinds us to remaining abilities. Every person is different and any intervention or treatment needs to reflect individual needs, desires and abilities. Dementia is progressive and life limiting so a palliative approach is required. Some medications may improve symptoms for some; however, at the current time, non-medical management and lifestyle adaptation are the principal means of support.

Development of interprofessional competencies for the client with dementia

The capabilities of both current and future practitioners need to be considered for two reasons: first, in terms of the environment, in which the care of clients with dementia is delivered; second, in terms of the number of clients with dementia, with an anticipated 20% increase in people with the disease in 10 years' time (Australian Bureau of Statistics, 2014). The development of interprofessional capabilities internationally is outlined in Chapter 3. By reviewing these developments, with a thorough literature review and consultation with practitioners and researchers, the following four interprofessional concepts or capabilities have therefore been highlighted as essential considerations:

1 Professional and personal knowledge – this capability looks at the practitioner as a whole, as well as the client, and recognises not only the professional knowledge that an individual brings to the situation but also life skills, empathy and personal experience.

2 Collaborative skills – this aspect is included in many of the other frameworks. It is particularly important in this context as the client is likely to have a wide range of health and social care needs to take into consideration as well as dementia. Family and carer perspectives on the client's welfare are also necessary and therefore the team should include the family and carers as well as the individual practitioners.

3 Evidence-based practice – this capability is required in all aspects of health care delivery. The health care team members working with a person with

dementia need to ensure that not only their professional skills and knowledge are based on the best evidence available, but that their work as a team is evidence based and their practice is consistantly of the highest standard.

4   Leadership skills – this capability within the team context and taking responsibility not only for one's own actions but those of the team as a whole is required now, and will increasingly be required in the future, in the care of the client with dementia.

By reviewing the latest research, and in collaboration with Dementia Training Study Centres throughout Australia, we derived the following additional four interprofessional concepts or capabilities for consideration in dementia care:

1   The journey of dementia – this capability requires the health care team to have the requisite knowledge, skills and attitudes that reflect an understanding of the medical, social, spiritual, emotional and cognitive complexities of the disease from onset to death spanning many years, while recognising that the person has experienced many more years without the disease before health care teams became involved.

2   Person- and relationship-centred care –this capability requires members of the health care team to recognise that the person living with dementia is not defined by their disease. Person- and relationship-centred care – which recognises human needs to connect with people and places, maintain existing relationships and build new ones, and engage in meaningful activity that encourages connection with the community – is an essential aspect of dementia care.

3   Environmental and cultural aspects – every person lives within social, cultural and physical environments that impact on a person's ability to form meaningful relationships and act in ways that reflect their **personhood**. This capability requires a member of the health care team to assess, analyse and modify the social, cultural and physical contexts in which a person with dementia lives. In addition, health care teams must be aware of and amend the social, cultural and physical impact of the health service delivery context on the person with dementia and their family.

> **Personhood**
> The state or fact of being an individual or having human characteristics and feelings.

4   Ethical concepts – clinical decisions are embedded in an array of ethical challenges and decisions; the choice between intervention options, allocation of resources, infringing autonomy, imposing burdens on some for the benefit of others – the list can be endless. Each situation is composed of a number of facts and values, and points of view affect choices and decisions individuals make. This capability requires health care teams to have a strong ethical framework

in which to work and the ability to use ethical reasoning to guide clinical decision making, often in pressured and time limited situations.

In the care of a client with dementia both the dementia and interprofessional capabilities are intricately interwoven. This is demonstrated in the following model.

Model of Interprofessional Practice and Education – Dementia

The structure of the Model of Interprofessional Practice and Education – Dementia (MIPPE-D) resembles a rope or cord, comprising eight strands that reflect the eight concepts or capabilities which require consideration for effective interprofessional dementia care (see Figure 1.1). By interweaving each strand with the others, the rope increases strength and durability. A missing strand weakens the rope and increases the risk of failure while under tension.

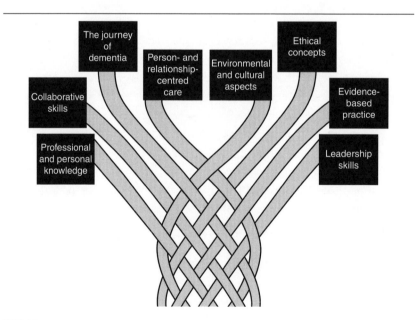

FIGURE 1.1   *The Model of Interprofessional Practice and Education – Dementia (MIPPE-D)*

The following chapters will explore these strands further and how they work together using case study examples.

Phoebe's life story

Case study

Dawn Forman and Heather Freegard

This case study has been adapted from a case study developed by the Western Australian Dementia Training Study Centre. Dementia Training Study Centres are funded by the Australian Government Department of Social Services. Visit http://www.dss.gov.au for more information.

This case study particularly highlights the journey of dementia, the importance of person- and relationship-centred care and the need for collaborative skills as taken from the MIPPE-D. Other aspects from the model are indicated just prior to each set of questions to help the reader.

Phoebe's life before dementia

Mary and Fred were married in a quiet ceremony in St Aloysius Anglican Church, Guildford, in March 1932. Fred was 48 and Mary 33. Fred, a quiet, shy man, was determined to have a good home before he married. His skills as a carpenter/furniture maker, and his frugal lifestyle, meant that he was able to purchase a block of land, and build and furnish a modest home during the Depression. He was also a skilled fiddle player and was in demand to play at local dances.

Mary was vivacious and outgoing. She left school at 14 and worked at the local telephone exchange. She was 18 when she married her sweetheart – a friend from childhood. She was a widow at 20, her husband dying as a result of a work injury (asphyxiation caused by the collapse of the side of the well that he was digging). She returned to her work at the telephone exchange and was relatively content with her lot in life. Her status as widow provided her with the freedom to engage in social activities denied to single women. She read avidly and widely – ancient history, politics and philosophy were her particular passions. She joined the local repertory club and became a skilled actress. One drama production required someone to play the role of a mute fiddle player and Fred was approached, and agreed. Mary and Fred met, fell in love and married.

The home established by Fred was at Guildford, at this time a small township near the river surrounded by market gardens and orchards. It linked to Perth via a railway and narrow road, and was a resting place for those travelling east from the city to the wheat belt and goldfields.

Phoebe was born at 3 am on 11 December 1937, the fourth child of Mary and Fred. She was born at home, her birth assisted by her maternal grandmother. She had two elder brothers – Jack Frederick (born 1933) and Stephen John (born 1935). Her elder sister, Joan Elizabeth (born 1936), lived just three months, contracting pertussis (whooping cough). The two boys were also very ill but recovered. The advice of the day was to have another child quickly as a means of overcoming the grief associated with the death of a child, so Phoebe was born just 10 months following Joan's death. There were no more children (as Mary was 40, and Fred 55).

Home was a happy place, full of laughter and music. Learning was valued and scholarly success was well regarded. All children were welcome in the carpentry workshop and learnt the skills and respect for tools from their father. As older parents, Fred and Mary encouraged conversation and debate at the dinner table. Phoebe, as the youngest child and only girl, felt very special and had a special bond with her father, often spending time in his presence in a companionable silence. From this secure place, the children were free to roam and explore their environment, and play with their friends, with one exception – they were forbidden from going into the town centre or railway station precincts alone. Mary wanted to protect her children from the many desperate strangers who were travelling as they sought work.

There was a shadow in the home. While unspoken, there was a sadness, especially within Mary. Several times each week, she could be found sitting quietly under the frangipani tree that had been planted in remembrance of Joan. When seen unawares, her body was drooped, her face slack, with tears silently rolling down her cheeks. On becoming aware that she was being observed, she would immediately brighten and make some excuse for her being there. 'Gosh, the heat has made me tired,' or 'I have a slight headache and thought the quiet would help it go away.' Phoebe always felt that her mother, while being loving and inclusive, also treated her with a reserve, and was both more protective and more demanding of academic excellence from her compared with her brothers.

The house and workshop were the hub of the repertory club activities, with friends and acquaintances coming and going. While the children were little, Mary did not take an active part in the repertory club, although she contributed by making and mending costumes, which she could do at home. Fred continued, happy to work backstage on set construction and props management. As the children grew up, they also became involved with front-of-house activities, handing out programs, ushering and assisting their parents in their respective chores.

Phoebe attended a small two-teacher primary school run by the State Education Department. Years 1–3 were in one classroom and Years 4–7 in the second. The family school years occurred during World War II, and the period of post-war construction. For the children, the war was an exciting backdrop and the theme for many mock war games where the brave Brits and Aussies defeated the Nazis and the Japs in the air, on the battlefield and on the seas. At the movies, newsreels of the day showed the patriotic and heroic deeds of the Allied Forces as they fought against the Nazis in Europe and the urgent need to stop the 'Yellow Peril' in their tracks before they reached Australian soil. Fred was too old to enlist and he became the surrogate father figure to many children in the district as he quietly attended to the many home maintenance tasks for the women whose husbands were away. Mary had to contend with some rationing of food and other daily resources. Otherwise the war had little impact on daily life.

After the war, some fathers did not return. Others returned wounded or emotionally scarred. Anger and resentment towards the Japanese, for their treatment of prisoners of war, and praise for the Americans, for finishing the war, was a common topic in social discussion and newspapers of the day.

Phoebe excelled at school academically and socially. She was a natural leader, sensitive to the needs of her fellow students. As a small school, with fewer than 70 students, all students were required to mix and interact with younger and older children, as well as those of their own age. The teacher would give individual attention to the older students in the classroom, and often relied on Phoebe to assist and supervise the younger students in class. Phoebe won a prestigious scholarship to further her education and, unlike the majority of her girlfriends, she continued to attend school to matriculation (Year 12). Going to high school was exciting and challenging, for the first time in her life mixing with others of similar intellectual capacity and interests. Teachers encouraged her abilities, treated her as an equal to the boys and challenged her to excel. Going to high school was also time-consuming and exhausting. Travel by train from Guildford to Perth Modern School in Subiaco was a slow and tedious journey by steam train, hot in summer and cold in winter. Phoebe often left home just as the sun was rising and arrived home after sunset. She was expected to take her share of the household chores and complete her homework. This left little time to maintain her old friendships and interests. However, she did continue with the repertory club on weekends.

Phoebe matriculated with distinction in English literature, European history, geography, chemistry and mathematics, and was offered a scholarship to the University of Western Australia. However, Phoebe chose a teachers' training college and, three years later, graduated as a primary school teacher. At 19, her first posting was to a small country town, teaching Years three and four. She shared a house with three other female teachers and became active in the local repertory club. There she met Joseph, then 25, the eldest son of a well-to-do wheat and sheep farmer.

Joseph (Joe) and Phoebe were married two years later and they set up a home together on the farm in a modest newly built house, 100 metres from the main house. The farm was large and prosperous, producing wheat and wool. Ten km of gravel road, and a further 800-metre entry road, separated the homestead from town. Joseph, the eldest child and only son, was destined to take over the farm from his father, in due course. His three younger sisters had married farmers and settled outside the district.

Joe and Phoebe were the perfect couple, well-liked, attractive and deeply in love. However, on the farm, away from public gaze, life was very different. Joe was a strict supervisor with high expectations of Phoebe's efforts both within the home and on the farm. He discouraged Phoebe from inviting friends to the farm and also from leaving the farm except for essential business. In addition to establishing the gardens, keeping the home spotless and providing well-cooked meals, Phoebe was required to drive the tractors, feed the stock and be a roustabout in the shearing shed. Even while pregnant, her workload did not decrease. At eight-months' pregnant she took the evening shift to make sure that the wheat crop was seeded before the rains came.

They had been married for three years when twins, Frances and Luke, were born. Tensions between Phoebe and Joe increased. Phoebe was no longer able to continue with all her farming chores, and Joe became angry with her for shirking her responsibilities and spoiling the children. He became very jealous of the attention Frances and Luke were given. Verbal abuse escalated to physical abuse directed towards Phoebe, made worse by Joe's increasing reliance on alcohol. Joe's parents were aware of Phoebe's increasing unhappiness but could not see their son's behaviour as contributing to the situation.

When the twins were six months old, Phoebe received a telephone call from Mary. Fred, now 78, had had a heart attack and was not expected to live. Phoebe, with the babies, rushed to Perth in time to say goodbye to her father and promise to take care of his Mary. Phoebe stayed in the family home with Mary in the weeks following Fred's death to support her mother, and assist her brothers in arranging the funeral and settling the estate.

Although this was a sad and busy time, Phoebe became less weary. It soon became apparent that Phoebe was loath to return to Joe and the farm. One evening she broke down and disclosed her unhappiness to her brother Stephen. He was appalled at Joe's behaviour, so he, with Mary and Jack, encouraged Phoebe to remain in the family home and live with her mother. Mary was experiencing shortness of breath and high blood pressure.

Joe was angry at Phoebe's desertion. During the acrimonious divorce proceedings, Phoebe was deemed to be 100% to blame for the breakdown of marriage and received no financial support. Because of their young age, the twins were allowed to remain with Phoebe.

With Mary's support with child care, Phoebe (who had been required to resign from the education department when she got married) sought employment. As a divorced woman, all she could find was part-time relief teaching.

Five years later, after a rapid decline, Mary died of cancer of the bowel and liver. To settle Mary's will, it was necessary to sell the family home. Phoebe used her part of the bequest to purchase a unit in Coolbellup. The suburb had a similar market garden–urban feel about it. Next to the small block of units, the Boden family, her Italian neighbours, lived on a large block and, in addition to providing Frances and Luke the experience of being part of a large extended family, also kept the small family generously provided with fresh vegetables, fruit and eggs. Phoebe continued her teaching and provided a stable home for herself, Frances and Luke. Phoebe was able to give maximum energy to parenting and work.

For the first time in her life, Phoebe had a period of self-efficacy and autonomy. The life of a single mother was difficult, although the rise of feminism, and changes to family law and social policy, were beginning to destigmatise the experience. The security of home ownership freed Phoebe of immediate financial worries. When her children started school, she was able to combine her roles as single mother and professional woman and increased her working hours. Phoebe became well-known for her in-school drama programmes for primary school children, especially in the areas of language development and social inclusion. Mrs Boden was a loved and reliable backstop on the rare occasions that Phoebe could not be at home on time.

When the twins were 13, Joe demanded that he have contact with the children. Reluctantly, Phoebe sent them to the farm for a two-week stay during the school holidays. Luke settled into the farming routine easily, with a natural talent for stock work. In his eyes, his father was an ideal role model. He wanted to stay. Phoebe and Joe finally agreed that Luke would finish school at agricultural college and on graduation return to the farm. From this point on, Phoebe and Frances saw little of Luke – the occasional affectionate visit, or warmly expressed messages on birthday and Christmas cards and rare phone calls.

Between Frances and Joe, there was an instant and deep antipathy. They did not get on at all; there was much bickering and arguing between them. At the end of the holiday period, Frances vowed never to go back to the farm. Joe disowned his daughter, happy that his son wanted to continue the family tradition on the farm.

Back in the city, Frances thrived, becoming a confident and competent young woman. At 18, when Phoebe was 43, she left home to attend university and live in shared accommodation.

Phoebe enjoyed living alone; she had a satisfying teaching career and spent her leisure time in repertory – and discovered the joy of travel. Her saving and holiday routine became established, embarking on a major trip abroad every three years – to India, Peru, Madagascar, Italy and Finland.

On retirement at 60, Phoebe planned to continue her travels to exciting and out-of-the-way places. Her health was good, rarely succumbing to coughs and colds, although having annoying bouts of urinary tract infections. She had become more sedentary, preferring to read in preparation for her next holiday and watch television. The degenerative changes in her shoulders, knees and hips, as a result of the heavy farm work, became bothersome. She still enjoyed eating and gained weight. When she went for her annual check-up with her GP, he warned her that she had developed hyperlipidaemia and encouraged her to exercise more and reduce her weight. He prescribed cholesterol-lowering medication and a mild analgesic to relieve joint pain, and discussed the possibility of hip replacement surgery in the future.

Phoebe continued to travel; now joining travel groups, and choosing less physically demanding destinations to accommodate her physical abilities. She found companionship among the other tour members and her extensive Christmas card list grew. For her 65th birthday, Frances gave her mother a computer as a means of managing her extensive social contacts and introduced her to email. Phoebe took to the new technology with enthusiasm and quickly became proficient at word processing and emailing.

Gradually her enthusiasm for travel and keeping in contact with friends waned. She lost her car no claim bonus following a series of minor but costly traffic incidents: running into the back of a Porsche at traffic lights; side swiping a four-wheel drive as she backed out of a parking bay; mistaking first gear for reverse and driving into a ditch; and driving over the speed limit on the freeway. Frances was called to reset her computer settings and demonstrate how to complete steps that Phoebe had previously done easily. She began to blame the computer for mistakes that occurred. Plans for her trip to New Zealand became complicated. She had difficulty choosing an itinerary, deposits were not confirmed. Her self-confidence waned. She frequently consulted her daughter, something she had rarely done previously.

Aspects of the MIPPE-D to consider when reviewing the case study so far and addressing the questions below are:

- the journey of dementia;
- person- and relationship-centred care.

Reflective questions

1 What is the significance of knowing and understanding the life history?
2 How can you help capture a person's history when they first come into care?
3 What are the key aspects of Phoebe's life which could impact on her care?

Case study ctd.

Early diagnosis of dementia

Mrs Boden, in great agitation, rang Frances late one afternoon. At first it was almost impossible to interpret her hurried, heavily accented Italian English. She got the gist of the story, reassured Mrs Boden and immediately drove to Phoebe's home. Phoebe had become disorientated in the stairwell at the back of the house and had fallen, bumping her head. Mrs Boden had heard Phoebe's distressed cries and came over to investigate. After assuring herself that Phoebe was not seriously hurt, she called an ambulance and Phoebe was taken to hospital to be assessed.

While Phoebe was in hospital following her fall, Frances went to Phoebe's home to collect some nighties. Frances noticed that the letter box had not been emptied for several weeks. Bills were unpaid and there was a large pile (Frances estimated at least four weeks' worth) of clothes and linen waiting to be laundered. As Frances opened the laundry door, her nostrils were assailed by the distinct odour of stale urine.

In hospital, Phoebe received a thorough medical and social assessment. She was diagnosed as having marked cognitive decline, probably mixed in aetiology with contributions from vascular dementia, and dementia of the Alzheimer's type, hyperlipidaemia, hypertension and bilateral osteoarthritis of hips, knees and shoulders.

When Phoebe returned home from hospital, the weekly home help and social access to a drop-in centre once each week arranged by the social worker began. With Phoebe's assent, Frances was appointed enduring power of attorney to allow her to manage her financial affairs. Phoebe appreciated the support of Frances and enjoyed the company of Hilary and John, the community support workers, who came to assist her with showering and house cleaning. She enjoyed less the drop-in centre, finding all the other members 'too old and deaf', but was amenable to continuing because she could help the others. All went well for six months.

There were several traumatic events in the following 12 months. The contract for providing community services was awarded to a different service organisation, resulting in both Hilary and John being transferred to other clients. Over several weeks, four different care workers were appointed but none stayed more than a week and they arrived at the house at different times. The lack of continuity upset Phoebe and she could not understand what was happening. She perceived that strangers were intruding into her house and expecting her to undress in front of them. She became very suspicious and, on one occasion, would not open the door to the care worker. To ensure her mother's safety and for reassurance, Frances visited her mother after work every evening. Eventually a consistent pattern was achieved and firm relationships were developed with the new care workers, and Frances and Phoebe felt safe again.

Next Phoebe became lost in the supermarket; the police were called when she became distressed and abusive to staff. On another occasion, she locked herself out of the unit and accused Mrs Boden of changing her door locks. When Frances called, there was no food in the house and Phoebe accused Frances of stealing her money. The Boden family, while being sympathetic, could no longer tolerate Phoebe's unpredictable behaviour.

Moving to a care facility

An emergency review was arranged and Phoebe was assessed as eligible for a place in a dementia-specific residential facility. With assessment in hand, Frances went about locating a suitable facility with a vacancy from the list of services provided by the social worker. Phoebe's resources allowed Frances to place Phoebe in a reputable facility that offered dementia-specific services. Three months' later, Phoebe left her long-time home and moved into Bradley Care House. Frances was unable to attend to her work commitments as well and claimed one month's special leave at short notice. While sympathetic to Frances' situation, her employer made it clear that her absence from work was very inconvenient.

The transition did not go smoothly. To make all the necessary arrangements – finding a suitable facility, attending to legal and financial matters, preparing Phoebe for the move, selecting furniture and belongings and finally settling her mother into her new abode – was exhausting for Frances. Luke arranged to bring his ute and moved the selected furniture into Bradley Care House while Frances dealt with the myriad decision-making and organisational tasks. Phoebe could participate in discussions and decisions about her care if the discussions were taken step by step, slowly, with reassurance and repeated information. Frances was required to make important decisions quickly and often the urgency of the situation resulted in hurried conversations with Phoebe. Phoebe became confused, anxious, suspicious and argumentative, exacerbating Frances' stress.

When everything was finally in order, Frances and Phoebe spent two days in a beachside cottage. The calm and change of scenery quickly settled Phoebe, and Frances had a brief respite to recharge her physical, emotional and cognitive batteries in preparation for the transition to come.

The following morning, Frances drove her mother to Bradley Care House where she was greeted warmly and shown to her room. She recognised her furniture and memorabilia, and felt comfortable. After a shared morning tea in Phoebe's room, Frances took her leave. The facility manager suggested to Frances that she let her mother settle in for a few days before visiting again, and reassured her that Phoebe would be fine and quickly settle in. Frances walked slowly to the car, opened the door, sat in the driver's seat, stared blankly ahead for a long minute and then burst into tears.

To meet Commonwealth requirements, staff were busy assessing and documenting Phoebe's care in support of the Aged Care Funding Instrument claim. All documentation was recorded in Phoebe's case notes.

Settling in

Phoebe did settle in. From the door of her room she could see the dining and sitting rooms and front foyer – all areas where residents, staff and family congregated. Phoebe enjoyed spending time with others, talking, walking and sometimes in companionable silence. Some residents she avoided: the male residents because they 'gave her the creeps'; those who were deaf because 'they can't have a conversation'; and Miriam who 'pours salt in her tea, walks into other people's rooms and continually asks people for the time because she is as mad as a cut snake'.

The lady in the adjacent room, Miss Meryl Falconer, also a retired teacher, became a firm friend. Phoebe entertained residents and staff with recitations of poetry, and monologues from well-known plays. Her imitations of Lady Bracknell from *The Importance of Being Earnest* caused much merriment.

Frances visited her mother twice each week. On Wednesday evenings, she dined with her mother and the other residents in the dining room, and then spent the evening with Phoebe in her room, reminiscing, reading mail and completing some small household tasks, such as mending or arranging the fresh flowers that she brought each week. Each Saturday, Phoebe would go out with Frances, sometimes to the shops or a drive but most often to Frances' home for a home-cooked meal, a potter in the garden and a quiet snooze. As the weeks passed, Frances noted that Phoebe no longer enjoyed her food. She declined cake, biscuits and other dry foods, preferring softer foods, and needed extra gravies, sauces and custards to enable her to swallow. Frances mentioned to the health care staff that Phoebe had always found it difficult to swallow pills, especially large capsules.

Aspects of the MIPPE-D to consider when reviewing the case study so far and addressing the questions below are:

- the journey of dementia;
- collaborative skills;
- environmental and cultural aspects.

Reflective questions

1 How could we use the knowledge of Phoebe's life to help to continue her meaningful life whilst in a new environment?
2 Which members of the health care team could be involved in assessing Phoebe at this stage?
3 How would you ensure that the members of the health care team collaborate effectively and work with Phoebe's family?

Case study ctd.

Phoebe did not particularly enjoy the social activities arranged within the facility, although she would generally agree to participate 'to help the others', with the exception of bingo, which she detested. She maintained her competitive spirit, and preferred to complete quizzes and word puzzles by herself rather than team up with residents with less ability. Her favourite pastime was walking in the gardens, which she tried to do each morning and afternoon in the company of Meryl. However, opportunities to do so were limited by external doors being locked to prevent some residents leaving the building, staff requiring Meryl and Phoebe to remain indoors to await the arrival of the GP and other health professionals, and set meal times.

She was allocated a small, raised garden bed to tend but, after three months, gave up because Mr Peters, another resident, helpfully 'weeded' all the newly planted seedlings and the gardener shifted the water hose connections so that Phoebe could not get water to her plants. Two days' later, the gardener cheerfully replaced the hose connections but, by then, the few remaining plants that Mr Peters had missed died. Phoebe missed doing the 'ordinary' things such as cooking, ironing and cleaning, although she happily relinquished grocery shopping, washing the laundry and vacuuming.

All in all, Phoebe had a lot of spare time on her hands, which she found increasingly difficult to use in a meaningful way. She became bored and restless, and began walking up and down the passages. Sometimes, she would misjudge the distance between herself and other residents and furniture, which meant that she often bumped into people and furniture. Some residents became fearful of her and others abusive of her perceived lack of respect. On two occasions, a resident fell to the floor, resulting in skin tears and general commotion as staff used a hoist to assist them from the floor. Phoebe herself became covered in bruises and skin tears on her forearms and shins. On two occasions, Phoebe and Meryl did take a walk outside independently. The first occasion went without incident and both women returned content. On the second occasion, Phoebe and Meryl were spotted by a staff member driving her car. They were several kilometres from Bradley House and attempting to cross a busy road. The staff member stopped her car and offered them a lift back home. Whilst not recognising the staff member, they willingly settled into the car and were pleased at the welcome reception on their return. Phoebe and Meryl were no longer permitted outside without supervision. Phoebe's agitation gradually increased as she tried to open the external doors and, finding them locked, started entering the rooms of other residents and berating them for being in 'her' room.

Aspects of the MIPPE-D to consider when reviewing the case study so far and addressing the questions below are:

- the journey of dementia;
- collaborative skills.

Reflective questions

1 What further amendments to a care plan would you now like to see put in place?
2 Who should be involved in the discussion at this stage?

Case study ctd.

Communication and language difficulties

One Friday afternoon, Phoebe bumped into a chair and slipped to the floor, bumping her left shoulder on the chair back. She said her shoulder hurt and began rubbing it. The senior supervisor – sure that there was no serious injury requiring an ambulance, but mindful that the weekend was fast approaching – called the registered nurse on duty: Melanie. Melanie assessed Phoebe and, while agreeing with the supervisor that there was no serious cause for concern, requested the doctor to visit. Phoebe's regular GP was unavailable and so the locum service was called. The senior supervisor rang Frances to advise her of the situation but Frances did not answer and the call went through to message bank.

The locum arrived at 5 pm, just as the residents and staff were readying themselves for the evening meal. Dr Lee was Chinese in appearance and carried a large medical bag in one hand and a stethoscope in the other. He had an imposing manner and spoke with a clipped accent. Melanie escorted Dr Lee to Phoebe's door. Both walked quickly and purposefully. Melanie knocked on the door and entered the room. Phoebe was seated in her armchair listening to the radio. Melanie turned off the radio, introduced the doctor and left to attend to the needs of other residents. Dr Lee matter-of-factly summarised why he had been called and simultaneously leant forward to examine her left shoulder, and asked her to remove her cardigan so that he could get a better look. Phoebe became very defensive, crossing her right arm across her body and shrinking into her chair, wincing as she moved. As Dr Lee persisted, she struck out with her right arm and yelled, 'Get away from me, you Jap.' Without a further word, Dr Lee straightened up, backed off, collected his bag and stethoscope, and left the room.

Hearing Phoebe's raised voice, the senior supervisor hurried down the corridor to investigate, meeting the doctor as he was closing Phoebe's door. In the office Dr Lee sat at the desk to write up his notes and prescription. Melanie apologised profusely, saying that Phoebe's extreme behaviour was completely out of character. Her GP, Dr Moyez, was Indian and she thought he was lovely. Dr Lee said tersely not to worry about it – it happened all the time. However, as he was unable to examine Phoebe thoroughly, all he could do was increase her analgesia.

Frances arrived just as Dr Lee was leaving. Then Melanie, who should have finished work two hours' previously, briefly updated Frances on the afternoon's events, grabbed her handbag and left. Frances went to her mother's room. When she arrived, her mother was calm and pleased to see her.

Aspects of the MIPPE-D to consider when reviewing the case study so far and addressing the questions below are:

- professional and personal knowledge;
- environmental and cultural aspects;
- evidence-based practice;
- leadership skills.

Reflective questions

1 Knowing Phoebe's history, what could explain her reaction?
2 What in Dr Lee's approach could have been done differently?
3 How should a health care professional have approached Phoebe and gained her confidence?
4 What could be done to improve the communication between members of the health care team?
5 What could have helped to respond or defuse this situation or even prevent it?
6 Why did Dr Lee say he could only prescribe more analgesics?

Case study ctd.

Phoebe aged 70

Phoebe celebrated her 70th birthday in the care home with family and the friends she had made in the home, including Miss Falconer, with whom she had become very close. Phoebe really seemed to enjoy the day. However, her enjoyment seemed short-lived as most days Phoebe now spent her time walking in the corridors and this was becoming increasingly aimless and slower. She could no longer make her own way to the dining or lounge areas, requiring reminding of the time and where to go. Her difficulty with swallowing worsened, now unable to chew solid foods and having difficulty using eating utensils. Other residents complained that her table manners were poor. She poured salt into her tea. She began wandering the corridors at night, disturbing the sleep of other residents. Miss Falconer passed away. Phoebe had lost her closest friend and companion in the facility.

Staff discussed with Frances and Luke the possibility of moving Phoebe into the high-care section of the facility where she would receive more care and supervision. Now that Miss Falconer had passed away, the children agreed that a move was appropriate.

Aspects of the MIPPE-D to consider when reviewing the case study so far and addressing the questions below are:

- environmental and cultural aspects;
- ethical concepts.

Reflective questions

1 What are the advantages and disadvantages of moving Phoebe at this time?
2 What can be done to make this transition as easy as possible?

Case study ctd.

Phoebe and all her own possessions were moved into the high-care section on Tuesday morning. Her room layout was similar to her previous room, which made reorientation easier for Phoebe. Her bathroom was to the left instead of the right, resulting in Phoebe entering the wardrobe in error.

Although Frances had met Melanie (one of Phoebe's nurses), she was relieved to have ongoing contact with Fiona, a member of staff who had known Phoebe (and herself) while in the hostel. Frances relied heavily on Fiona during the transition for emotional support and as an information source and go-between with staff. As Dr Moyez had recently left the practice Dr Bennett became Phoebe's GP.

Aspects of the MIPPE-D to consider when reviewing the case study so far and addressing the questions below are:

- environmental and cultural aspects;
- leadership skills;
- evidence-based practice.

Reflective questions

1 What does the research say about changing the accommodation of a person with dementia?
2 What could the family and the health care team do to improve Phoebe's life at this stage?

Case study ctd.

Three weeks after Phoebe's relocation, a family meeting was planned. Frances and Luke met with Melanie, Dr Bennett and Fiona.

Melanie led the meeting, asking each member to provide Frances and Luke with a brief summary of Phoebe's situation and the reasons why the decision was made to move Phoebe to high care. Dr Bennett noticed Luke's increasing discomfort and distress as Melanie was speaking. On asking whether Luke had anything he wished to say, Luke suggested that this was not the mother he knew, that it was unfair that her life should be limited and, like a loved animal on the farm, she should be put out of her misery. At this point, Frances became upset and accused Luke of being insensitive and cruel.

Acting as peacemaker, Dr Bennett suggested that both points of view indicated a strong commitment to Phoebe's welfare, and desire for a comfortable and meaningful life for their mother. Once the emotion had calmed down, Dr Bennett suggested that a good way forward was to prepare an advance care plan, explaining that, as Phoebe had been unable to prepare an advance care directive, it was up to the family, with the support of the team, to determine what could/should be done and how Phoebe should be treated.

Frances asked what Phoebe's future was and what was likely to happen. Dr Bennett explained that Phoebe was now in the advanced stages of dementia and, while impossible to estimate the length of time, she would eventually die. Luke asked what the dying would be like. Dr Bennett explained that everyone was different but emphasised that, with the good care provided by Melanie and staff, she would be well cared for and comfortable, which was why their input into what Phoebe valued and what should happen was really important.

Dr Bennett inquired whether Phoebe had expressed how she would like to be treated in the event of her not being able to make her wishes known. How did she view life? Did she think about dying and death? Luke explained that, as he had pretty much left home at 13, he could not say for sure but he was sure that she would not want to live like this, like a vegetable.

Frances described her mother as a determined person who always stuck things through to the end, never giving up. She was always able to find something enjoyable or amusing in any situation. Like now, she liked to be by the window and see the garden and watch the birds. But she would hate to be a burden on others and think she was being a nuisance.

Dr Bennett appreciated these insights and the emotional stresses experienced by both Luke and Frances, suggesting that they and the staff could respect Phoebe's values in the way she was cared for to make sure she lived a comfortable life for the time she had left.

Frances was worried that her mother did not seem to be eating properly and suggested she must be hungry. She had heard of people having their food fed directly into their tummy. Melanie explained that PEG feeding could be done but it was not a practice carried out at Bradley Care House. If that was what they wanted, Phoebe would need to be transferred to another facility and help would be provided to do that if required. Melanie explained that Phoebe was not as active as she used to be and didn't need the amount of food she used to eat. Her weight had been stable since she arrived and, now that she was on a liquid diet and staff were taking the time to help her eat, she was enjoying her food more.

Dr Bennett supported Melanie's comments saying that inserting a PEG was an invasive procedure, and not without risks and complications. There was also some discussion about whether having a PEG actually helped people with dementia. Frances indicated that she did not want her mother to have to go to hospital to have a PEG fitted as she felt that the change in environment would confuse her mum even more. Dr Bennett therefore asked whether, if Phoebe was to have any other ill health issues, the family would still prefer her to be looked after in the care home rather than be taken to hospital. The family agreed. Dr Bennett then gently indicated that, while Phoebe was well at the moment, she was conscious that, as with all the people in the home, Phoebe could have a severe stroke or heart attack. She therefore recommended that, as Phoebe was quite weak, she did not feel it would be in Phoebe's interest for attempts to be made to resuscitate her. Frances broke into tears at this point but through those tears said that she agreed. This was noted in Phoebe's medical notes and members of the health care team were informed.

Aspects of the MIPPE-D to consider when reviewing the case study so far and addressing the questions below are:

- environmental and cultural aspects;
- leadership skills;
- ethical concepts.

Reflective questions

1 Why do you think Dr Bennett tried to gain the agreement of the family at this stage?
2 What are the ethical issues in making such suggestions?
3 Could more have been done to ensure that all the health care team were informed?

End-of-life care

Phoebe continued to lose interest in her food, lost weight, became bed ridden and lost all interest in communicating. While the staff did what they could to encourage Phoebe to eat, even her favourite trifle was refused. Frances visited regularly and gradually came to realise that her Mum was nearing the end of her life. Frances met regularly with Dr Bennett and members of the health care team, all of whom made every effort to make Phoebe comfortable. The care staff cleaned Phoebe's mouth, when eventually she would not take fluid or food, and turned her regularly to ensure that she did not get pressure sores. They ensured that, when she was washed, her skin was moisturised with her favourite perfumed cream,

Case study ctd.

her hair was combed neatly and they talked to her all the time they were with her. When warm enough, the window was opened so that she could hear the sounds of children playing in the school nearby, which she used to love.

Frances talked things through with her brother and together they started to talk about their mum's life and how they thought she would like to be remembered when the time came.

Early one morning, a member of staff from the care home phoned Frances to say that Phoebe's breathing pattern had changed and advised her to come to the home. Frances noticed that Phoebe seemed to be really struggling with each intake of breath, her eyes seemed to be fixed on one corner of the room and Frances was told that her blood pressure was also very low. Luke also came to be with his mum and, as they sat with her, Phoebe passed away. Phoebe was 72 when she died.

Aspects of the MIPPE-D to consider when reviewing the case study so far and addressing the questions below are:

- the journey of dementia;
- collaborative skills;
- professional and personal knowledge.

Reflective questions

1 How has Phoebe's story made you feel, not only as a professional, but also as a person?
2 How has Phoebe's story changed the way you will see a person with dementia?
3 How do you think the health care team feel as they let the family say goodbye to Phoebe?
4 How can the team now best support each other and Phoebe's family members?

Take the opportunity to reread this case study

We would like you to note your responses to these questions now and to reread this case study when you have read the other chapters of this book.

1 What are you thinking now? How has this changed from when you first read the case study?
2 What will you do when you meet a person with dementia?

Conclusion

This chapter has outlined the development of interprofessional competencies and capabilities, and how these combine with the competencies needed when carers and professionals are working with individuals with dementia. It is the combination of these capabilities, with the constant focus on the needs of the individual, which is crucial in practice. The following chapters will use case study examples to explore this further. We recommend that the case study at the end of this chapter is read after Chapter 1 and again when you have read the full book or completed your program, as we believe that you will notice different things in the case study the second time and may address the questions in a different way.

Self-directed learning activities

1   The MIPPE-D Framework has been derived from research and practice internationally. Does it cover all the aspects of the capabilities you feel are needed in practice?
2   A strong feature of the MIPPE-D is the way in which the strands intertwine and that too strong a focus on one aspect would mean that the care of the individual may not be appropriate. Do you think that is true?
3   How can these concepts and capabilities be measured in practice?

References

Ajjawi, R. & Higgs, J. (2008). Learning to reason: A journey of professional socialisation. *Advances in Health Sciences Education: Theory and practice*, 13(2): 133–50. doi: 10.1007/s10459–006–9032–4

Atkinson, M., Wilkin, A., Stott, A., Doherty, P. & Kinder, K. (2002). *Multi agency working: A detailed study*. Berkshire: National Foundation for Educational Research.

Australian Bureau of Statistics. (2014). Retrieved 30 March 2015 from http://www.abs.gov.au/ausstats/abs@.nsf/Lookup/3222.0main+features32012%20%28base%29%20to%202101

Barr, H. (2002). *Interprofessional education: Today, yesterday and tomorrow*. London: CAIPE.

Dahlgren, M., Richardson, B. & Sjostrom, B. (2004). Professions as communities of practice. In J. Higgs, B. Richardson & M. Dahlgren (eds) *Developing practice knowledge for health professionals* (pp. 71–88). Edinburgh: Butterworth Heinemann.

Goldenberg, D. & Iwasiw, C. (1993). Professional socialisation of nursing students as an outcome of a senior clinical preceptorship experience. *Nurse Education Today,* 13: 3–15.

Higgs, J., Andresen, L. & Fish, D. (2004). Practice knowledge – its nature, sources and contexts. In J. Higgs, B. Richardson & M. Dahlgren (eds) *Developing practice knowledge for health professionals* (pp. 51–69). Edinburgh: Butterworth Heinemann.

Johnsson, M.C. & Hager, P. (2008). Navigating the wilderness of becoming professional. *Journal of Workplace Learning,* 20(7/8): 526–36. doi: 10.1108/13665620810900346

Regehr, G. & Eva, K.W. (2007) Self-assessment, self-direction, and the self-regulating professional clinical orthopaedics and related research. *Clinical Orthopaedics and Related Research,* 449: 34–8. doi: 10.1097/01.blo.0000224027.85732.b2

Smith, R.A. & Pilling, S. (2007). Allied health graduate program – supporting the transition from student to professional in an interdisciplinary program. *Journal of Interprofessional Care,* 21(3): 265–76. doi: 10.1080/13561820701259116

World Health Organization (1978). *Guidelines for evaluating a training programme for health personnel.* Geneva: WHO.

2 The journey of dementia

Heather Freegard and Dimity Pond

Learning outcomes

1 Discuss the course of the disease from health to illness to death.

2 Discuss the importance of acknowledging the social, emotional and spiritual aspects of a person living with dementia.

3 Discuss the significance of the person's life lived before the onset of dementia.

4 Consider the impact of the journey of dementia on family and friends.

Key terms

● Alzheimer's disease

● dementia

● neurocognitive disorder (NCD)

● personality

Introduction

The journey of **dementia** can be described as follows:

● something is not right;
● diagnosis;
● course;
● transitions;
● end of life;
● life stories;
● the family experience.

Mace and Rabins (1981) made four connected statements about dementia:

1 there is damage to the brain;
2 the person is still there;

Dementia
Dementia is now referred to as a neurocognitive disorder (NCD) (American Psychiatric Association, 2013), that is, the result of chronic or progressive damage to the brain.

3 the family is also affected;

4 there are things we can do.

This chapter will expand on the first three statements and allude to the last.

As health or care professionals, we should always remember that people have lived 60 or 70 years before the onset of dementia – it does not define them. Each of us comes in and out of people's lives in just this small portion. Really we might be a bit important but in the totality we are just a small-bit player.

There is damage to the brain

Each individual is defined by actions taken or not taken, that is, behaviour, evaluated against social values and context. Some behaviour may be considered quirky or unusual, amusing, annoying, tolerated or admired. Some may be considered sufficiently different or out of character to indicate intervention by medical, legal, spiritual or educative authorities to bring the behaviours into acceptable norms. Some behaviour engenders distress, pity, fear or disgust to such a degree that removal from society, temporarily or permanently, into the control of experts, is the best way to keep the individual and society safe. The challenge for individuals and communities is to determine at what point a quirk or change in behaviour goes beyond annoying or tolerable and becomes a problem for the person, their family and friends or the community. There is no clear definition of 'normal' behaviour. This is the challenge presented by a **neurocognitive disorder (NCD)**, or dementia.

> **Neurocognitive disorder (NCD)**
> Neurocognitive disorder is an umbrella term to describe a collection of disease processes that cause different sequences of brain damage, and variations in appearance and severity of symptoms (American Psychiatric Association, 2013).

NCDs are the result of chronic or progressive damage to the brain. To most health professionals, this is an obvious statement of truth. However, it is the changed and changing behaviour and actions of people that provide the external evidence for the changing brain, and changing behaviour can be interpreted in many ways. In the beginning, the changes of behaviour are often subtle and insidious in nature, and easily ignored or explained away as a normal part of ageing or a reflection of the person's **personality**, or a natural reaction to stress or changed circumstances. It is virtually impossible to determine when the disease began. As behaviours become more concerning, other explanations, based on deep cultural or religious beliefs, may emerge; for example, normal ageing and response to getting older,

> **Personality**
> Personality is made up of the characteristic patterns of thoughts, feelings and behaviours that make a person unique. It arises from within the individual and remains fairly consistent throughout life.

madness, the invasion of angry spirits, an expression of God's wrath, karma or atonement for sins. These different understandings of the causes influence the quality of relationships with family and friends; how, or whether, they continue to be part of the community; and the nature of support and treatment received.

Major NCD (dementia) is a difficult diagnosis to make. There is no one test that will tell us whether a person could be accurately diagnosed with this disorder. Part of the reason is that the disease is a cluster of symptoms and each symptom could have a number of different causes. Such causes include delirium, depression, drug side effects and other physical illnesses causing alterations to the brain (e.g. brain tumour, increased pressure in the brain). To reach the diagnosis, these other causes need to be excluded, and that may take both multiple tests and some considerable time. Another problem is that dementia itself is not one disease but may be caused by many different processes. So we have vascular dementia, **Alzheimer's disease** and so on: all dementia but with different pathological processes to be identified.

Alzheimer's disease

Alzheimer's disease is the most common form of major neurocognitive disorder. It was first described by Dr Alois Alzheimer in 1907 as he found particular changes on post-mortem brain examination (American Psychiatric Association, 2013).

A diagnosis based on thorough expert investigation is relatively rare. The process is resource intensive, takes time – measured in months rather than weeks or days – and requires the expertise and collaboration of many experienced health professionals. Many Australians with dementia never receive a diagnosis, or the diagnosis is made in the later stages (Kitwood, 1993). For many others, the diagnosis is given without full investigation and, occasionally, people who have treatable causes of behavioural change are labelled with dementia. Possible reasons to explain this situation are many. For example, the person may be unaware that there is anything wrong and resist attempts to visit their GP or specialist; the family may resist the possibility of neurocognitive decline; the GP may not be able to observe any significant changes or listen closely to the family member in a short consultation; confidentiality concerns may mean that the GP does not discuss the patient with the relatives and therefore misses vital diagnostic information; or access to appropriate services may be limited.

A diagnosis of dementia is a two-edged sword. Knowing that there is a disease process affecting behaviours can be an enormous relief to the person and their families, struggling to understand and support each other. As with all diagnoses of a life limiting nature, there is time and opportunity to make informed decisions and plans to manage the future. Access to appropriate services and support groups, such as respite, counselling and home help, becomes available, and the marshalling of informal support from family, friends or neighbours is possible. On the other hand, there is still much stigma associated with cognitive loss and behavioural changes so that the person and the carer may experience social isolation and lose hope. The course of the disease is unpredictable and, as with many chronic and degenerative diseases, planning for the future can be challenging.

The living experience of the person with dementia is often overlooked. This is because the focus is on the losses associated with the disease and the resources needed to support the person and their family.

The person is still there

Dementia is generally associated with older age although this is not always the case. It is now better recognised that dementia can also occur in a person's forties and fifties, or occasionally even younger. Whether in their forties, fifties, sixties or seventies, the person living with dementia has had many decades of life experience. They have been a 'person without dementia' far longer than a person living with dementia. Such life experience builds on natural talents and personality, and provides opportunities to develop skills, knowledge, attitudes, assets and relationships. These resources influence resilience and this in turn affects their response to the challenges of dementia. As described below, Kitwood (1989) pioneered an approach that incorporates these factors into each person's care.

Philosophers across the ages have debated the question of what makes a human a person, especially in the context of how it makes humans different from other animals. Almost universally these definitions have included some reference to the ability to reason and to remember. (Descartes, 1644: *'cogito ergo sum'* [I think therefore I am]). Therefore, it is argued by some that a person who cannot, or has lost the abilities to, remember and reason is no longer a person. Being a non-person can mean that their rights, such as the right to freedom of association or retention of property, are no longer valid. Kitwood (1989) described this as 'malignant social psychology'.

Nancy Mace (Mace & Rabins, 1981) and Tom Kitwood (1989) were early advocates that a person is not, nor should be, defined by their disease. Kitwood's famous equation 'SD = P + B + H + NI +SP' succinctly explains that the clinical manifestations of the neurological impairment, or symptoms of dementia (SD) were more than the neurological impairment (NI) alone. The person's personality (P), their life history (background) (B), health status (H), and the social environment and the degree to which the person's abilities are fostered and limitations supported (SP – social psychology) can exacerbate or ameliorate the effects of brain damage (Kitwood, 1993). Kitwood argues that, while personality and biography cannot be altered, and the neurological impairment is either chronic or progressive in nature, it is possible to ensure that a person's overall health and welfare can be promoted so that a life of good quality can be experienced throughout the trajectory of dementia.

Nolan et al. (2004) expanded Kitwood's work and proposed that the social psychology around each person is expressed in relationship with others. To be truly fulfilling and empowering of personhood, the relationship should be reciprocal and the nature of connection between person, family, carer staff and health professionals should all be addressed. This further strengthens the notion that the person living with dementia is an active participant in their life, not just a passive recipient.

The family is also affected

Not all families have the skills and knowledge to support the person. Not all relationships are cordial. Family members can be emotionally close but geographically separated and vice versa.

Family members can be affected by many factors; for example, a sense of familial duty, guilt associated with not coping or shame associated with a family member demonstrating symptoms of dementia. Families are often torn between competing needs: the need to seek help, a feeling that they should be able to cope, and a lack of knowledge about how to go about getting assistance. There may be family arguments about whether or how help should be accessed. Overwhelmingly, the majority of carers are female, and caring responsibilities often result in loss of full-time work, and additional financial and time stressors. In Australia, for example, women represent 70% of primary carers (Australian Bureau of Statistics, 2012). Women may also be caught between the needs of caring for a relative with dementia and those of other family members, especially teenage children. Often families regard the use of services as a last resort.

As families are different, so are their methods of decision making. The responsibility for deciding about these issues will differ from family to family and may not be obvious to care providers. Sometimes decisions are made along gender lines with the 'man' of the family having the ultimate say, but often there are subtle pressures brought to bear, which may not be obvious to the outsider. Once services are brought in, families differ in the way they negotiate with service providers or non-providers. As dementia progresses, decisions about placement in residential aged care will need to be made, and this will involve another set of complex family decisions. Often these also involve financial matters, and the family members who negotiate with financial institutions are likely to be different from the ones who negotiate with home services.

These decisions are made more difficult by a number of layers of bureaucracy that must be negotiated. It is often not clear to families that they can't just place their relative in a nursing home In Australia, they need an aged care assessment team (ACAT) assessment first, which may take many weeks. Other countries have a variety of first call services, almost all of which would require some assessment process. Dealing with government departments and processes carries its own set of challenges, which may make the task of caring more onerous. Often it is not obvious to families what is available and they may not be easily able to articulate what they need either. In the early stages of the journey, particularly, it is often 'hit and miss' whether a family carer accesses particular services. Care providers themselves are not necessarily familiar with all the services available; it is a specialised area.

The work of accessing services for assessment is not only that of networking and using sources of information and support. It also involves sheer physical effort. Family and carers may need to travel some distance, perhaps by public transport, and penetrate the corridors of office buildings to find the right person to assist them. Such carers themselves are often elderly and this kind of work is a particular challenge in those cases. Even for younger carers, the work of visiting government departments may need to be prioritised with competing demands around family and other aspects of the caring role.

There are things we can do

There are many things that can be done to help people living with dementia and their families through this difficult time. Primary care professionals should remember that the journey is not clear to those who have never travelled it before and that directions are needed along the way. Often it is helpful to map out what might lie ahead as time goes on; for example, to mention early on that many families find it necessary to bring in assistance, to obtain respite care and to place their relative in residential care eventually. Common problems encountered by people with dementia should be mentioned: the tendency to suffer from delirium when physically unwell, the problems associated with loss of cognitive capacities, and the loss of physical as well as mental capacity. At some point, it is important that the family is told about the terminal nature of the disease. The health professional may do this at intervals, and perhaps repeatedly give out information and brochures about how to bring in assistance, obtain respite, and so on as required. Remember that the whole primary care team is working in this way and information may come at a critical moment from another team member.

It is helpful, in this process, for the family to work through some advance care planning, where they discuss options ahead of time and preferably with the input of the person living with dementia, if they are able. This makes life immensely easier for the family at critical junctures. For example, it might be decided relatively early on that, if the person living with dementia becomes doubly incontinent, then it would be reasonable to move to residential aged care. When this possibility becomes a sad fact, it is helpful to have had this discussion and be on the same page as a family about it. As this process evolves, various legal documents should also be completed, including the will, power of attorney and an advance care directive particularly aimed at the terminal phases of the disease.

Care providers should also remember that a comprehensive approach to assessing any problems that the person may have is preferable (Garratt & Pond, 2014). As well as purely physical problems, the care provider should pay attention to the need to explain as they go along, so that the person living with dementia and the carer can understand what is happening. Any change in functional ability should be noted and any new needs that the person or family may have as a result should be addressed. Strengths, such as retained functions and strong family support systems, should be acknowledged and built upon. The emotional health of both the person living with dementia and the carer should be considered at all times and action taken if there is a need to address depression or anxiety.

Self-help and consumer/carer groups – such as the local Alzheimer's support group (see Alzheimer's Australia (https://www.fightdementia.org.au/), the US Alzheimer's Association (http://www.alz.org) or the UK Alzheimer's Society (http://www.alzheimers.org.uk/)) – may be invaluable in assisting carers and consumers. These organisations offer a range of services; for example, telephone counselling services, a library, various groups, including education and support groups, and advocacy for people living with dementia and their carers.

Conclusion

Dementia is a terminal illness. As the terminal phase of the illness approaches, providers should consider a palliative approach to care. What does this involve?

According to the World Health Organization (n.d.):

> Palliative care is an approach that improves the quality of life of patients and their families facing the problem associated with life-threatening illness, through the prevention and relief of suffering by means of early identification and impeccable assessment and treatment of pain and other problems, physical, psychosocial and spiritual.

This means that the care provider will aim to relieve or palliate symptoms but is not necessarily aiming at a cure at this stage. Specific issues around pain, nutrition, hydration and antibiotics will need to be considered, always with the comfort of the person living with dementia in mind. Discussion between the family and the health care provider can assist with many of these issues. Usually admission to an acute care service in the terminal phases is not advisable (Abbey, 2006) as it causes distress to the person living with dementia and the family, and achieves no purpose in terms of quality, or indeed significant increase in the length, of life for the person living with dementia.

Self-directed learning activities

The following case studies and questions will help you consider these aspects further.

Case study

Rose was looking after her husband, Jim, in his 80s and suffering from mild-to-moderate dementia. She adamantly denied the need for any assistance when this was raised by Jim's doctor on several occasions, and even refused to take the phone number for the community care services. Some six months later, Rose spoke to the GP reproachfully. She said that her physiotherapist had told her that the community service providers would be helpful and had given her their number. Rose said that a nice lady from community care had been out and now she was accessing services that made life a lot easier for her and her husband, Jim.

Reflective questions

1 What might Rose have been thinking and feeling when the question of the aged care assessment team was first raised?
2 What might she have been thinking and feeling six months later, when she saw the physiotherapist?
3 Are external things, such as her husband's behaviour, likely to have changed in that time? Might any family dynamics have changed?
4 How might the GP best respond to the tone of reproach in her voice?
5 Is it appropriate for the physiotherapist to have given her the number of the community service providers? Is there anything else the physiotherapist might have done? Should the physiotherapist have contacted the GP?

Younger onset dementia: Rural area

Case study

Jack, aged 52, had run a small motor mechanic business in a rural town for many years. He lived slightly out of town and, together with his wife, bred sheep on a small holding. His wife also did the books for the business.

Over recent years, the business had slipped downhill, and many previously loyal customers started to take their vehicles to a slightly more distant larger town. Jack blamed this on the attractions of the larger place but, when questioned by his wife, appeared indifferent to the implications for the family finances.

In recent months, Jack hurt his back while servicing a vehicle. The GP advised some physiotherapy, so he started to attend the newly arrived physiotherapist in the town. She worked part time from home.

After about six sessions, the physiotherapist asked to see Jack and his wife together. She explained that she was concerned that Jack was not doing the exercises the way he was asked to. She said that it seemed to her that Jack was having difficulty understanding what was required. Despite Jack blustering that he just 'wasn't interested', she pointed out that, when he did the exercises with her, he felt quite a lot better but then he didn't follow up on doing them at home. Jack's wife, Anne, said that she had no idea that exercises had been prescribed. She promised to work with Jack to remind him to do them.

This worked for a few weeks but then Anne raised with Jack and the physiotherapist the difficulty he seemed to be having getting organised to do the exercises and also remembering them. Anne said that this was not the Jack she knew and told him that it was high time he saw the GP about this. She said that he was too young to have memory problems and the whole thing needed sorting out. The physiotherapist was very supportive of this approach and wrote a brief note outlining the problem for the GP.

Despite this letter, the GP was inclined to dismiss the problem when it was first raised. He stated that the physiotherapist was young and full of funny ideas from the university, and that Jack was too young to have memory problems. But Anne was persistent and Jack said that he would be happy to have some tests 'just to settle her down'. The GP asked his practice nurse to administer a cognitive function screening test (see SMMSE in Appendix), and ordered some blood tests and a brain computerised tomography (CT) scan for Jack. Jack needed to go to a larger place for the CT scan, a round trip of about 200km, and this took over a week to organise. In the meantime, the practice nurse discussed the results of the screening test with the GP. She said she was surprised at how many errors Jack had made and was concerned that there was in fact something wrong. She said that there was no obvious reason, such as distraction or lack of concentration, for Jack to have scored poorly.

On the review visit, the GP noted that the blood tests and scan were all normal but that Jack's performance on the screening test was significantly poorer than would be expected, and in fact in the dementia range. He discussed with Jack and his wife that there were indeed problems with Jack's memory and that he would need further testing through a specialist. This entailed another distant visit and resulted in a firm diagnosis of younger onset dementia (YOD).

The following year or two were turbulent ones in Jack and Anne's life. Anne had to take over the reins of closing down the business and persuading her husband that he should not continue to test drive customers' cars. She uncovered a chaotic mess of papers and receipts in the office, and went through these to organise them for taxation purposes. She gradually took on more and more of the household duties too, including the outside duties, as Jack's dementia was marked by significant apathy and he seemed to lack initiative to get up and go. She sold off a lot of the sheep and downsized the property. She also investigated the possibility of a sickness benefit for Jack, which took considerable time and effort, particularly as the Centrelink office did not appear to understand dementia in a younger person and questioned the diagnosis. They were also keen to rehabilitate Jack for different work but he was not capable of this as his dementia was following a rapidly progressive course.

Fortunately, the GP referred Anne to Alzheimer's Australia, which runs a key worker program to support people living with YOD. The key worker – Michelle – visited Jack and Anne from the large town closest to them and then kept in regular contact over the phone. Anne found this support invaluable as she sought to negotiate the complex maze of services and bureaucratic hurdles.

Jack passed away about five years after diagnosis. The last two years of his life were spent in a local residential care facility. This was not ideal as he was surrounded by people two or three decades older than him, and mostly women, but that was all that was available close to home.

Reflective questions

1 YOD affects people aged less than 65 years. What particular barriers might these people have to diagnosis?
2 Jack was first identified as having a problem by the physiotherapist. How common might this be? Did the physiotherapist behave appropriately in discussing the matter with Jack and his wife?
3 What additional costs might the rural setting have placed on Jack and his wife in obtaining diagnostic, assessment and support services?
4 Given that people living with YOD are often working, what particular additional burdens are placed on the carer?
5 Are you aware of any particular services for YOD? How should residential care respond best to this challenge?

References

Abbey, J. (2006). Palliative care and dementia. *Alzheimer's Australia*. Scullin, ACT: Alzheimer's Australia.

Australian Bureau of Statistics. (2012). *Disability, Ageing and Carers, Australia: Summary of Findings, 2012*. Document 5. Retrieved 22 February 2015 from http://www.abs.gov.au/ausstats/abs@.nsf/Lookup/5968BE956901DD79CA257D5700 1F4D89?opendocument

Descartes, R. (1644). Principia philosophiae. In J. Cottingham, R. Stoothoff, D. Murdoch & A. Kenny (trans and eds) *The philosophical writings of Descartes (1984–91)*, vol. 1. Cambridge: Cambridge University Press.

Garratt, S. & Pond, D. (2014). Person-centred comprehensive geriatric assessment. In R. Nay, S. Garratt & D. Fetherstonhaugh *Older people: Issues and innovations in care* (4th edn). Chatswood, NSW: Elsevier.

Kitwood, T. (1989). Brain, mind and dementia: With particular reference to Alzheimer's disease. *Ageing and Society*, 9: 1–15. doi: 10.1017/S0144686X00013337

Kitwood, T. (1993). Person and process in dementia. *International Journal of Geriatric Psychiatry*, 8(7): 541–5. doi:10.1002/gps.930080702

Mace, N.L. & Rabins, P.V. (1981). *The 36-hour day: A family guide to caring for people who have Alzheimer disease, related dementias, and memory loss* (5th edn). Baltimore, MD: Johns Hopkins University Press.

Nolan, M.R., Davies, S., Brown, J., Keady, J. & Nolan, J. (2004). Beyond person-centred care: A new vision for gerontological nursing. *Journal of Clinical Nursing*, 13: 45–53. doi:10.1111/j.1365–2702.2004.00926.x

World Health Organization. (n.d.). Definition of palliative care. Retrieved 26 August 2014 from http://www.who.int/cancer/palliative/definition/en/

National and international perspectives: Interprofessional education and collaborative practice

3

Dawn Forman

Learning outcomes

1. Discuss the drivers and imperatives for changing the way health care is provided.
2. Define interprofessional education and collaborative practice.
3. Discuss how interprofessional education and practice can respond to the imperatives and drivers in changing health contexts.
4. Discuss the relevance of interprofessional education and collaborative practice in the context of dementia care.

Key terms

- collaborative practice (CP)
- integrated approach
- interprofessional education (IPE)

Introduction

Many factors have precipitated increased interest in **interprofessional education (IPE)** and collaborative practice (CP). Demographic changes, in particular an ageing population and increased incidence of long-term health issues, require health care teams to work with people with complex care needs. New

Interprofessional education (IPE)
Interprofessional education occurs when two or more professions learn with, from and about each other to improve collaboration and the quality of care (http://www.caipe.org.uk/about-us/defining-ipe/). When students from two or more professions learn about, from and with each other to enable effective collaboration and improve health outcomes (WHO, 2010).

models of care and technological advances in diagnosis, treatment and rehabilitation practice require specialised knowledge to provide appropriate, safe and cost effective services. And, despite increasing university places for health professionals, the demand for qualified health professionals continues to exceed supply.

This chapter will look at the origins of IPE internationally, and the health care environment in which dementia care is to be provided, and ask: What is it? How was it developed? Why do we need it? What does it look like?

Drivers for changing the way health care is provided

In 2012, Health Workforce Australia published documentation looking to the future of what would be required for the health workforce in 2025. It articulated the need to develop a health workforce that would work towards new models of health care and, therefore, the need to develop new models of education and training. However, this concept is not new. Indeed Flexner (1910) advocated the need to transform medical education, shifting from an idiosyncratic apprenticeship model to a more rigorous systematic biomedical and educational approach.

Whilst Flexner is recognised as being key, at that time, to the transformation within the medical and health care curriculum, it was a report published by the World Health Organization (WHO) in 1978 that emphasised the need to ensure that health professionals would work together and gain appropriate competencies (see pp. 11–12, Chapter 1, for the quote from this report). The global need to constantly renew and review health care curricula can be traced to this time. However, developing a curriculum to facilitate what we now term as 'interprofessional education' has been slow in its inception and development.

Tope (1996) provided a review of IPE internationally and indicated that 'despite an intensive search, very little literature was found to describe interdisciplinary (interprofessional) activities in either Australia or New Zealand.'

Yet IPE has been a key agenda within government policies internationally for the past 30 years. Many recent reviews of health care systems in the UK (The King's Fund, 2011), Australia (Garling, 2008) and internationally (West,

Patera & Carsten, 2009) point to the need for new interprofessional models of health service delivery into the future. Equally these reports emphasise the impact of demographic trends in which there is an increasing ageing population and a decrease in the number of health professionals available to work in aged care environments.

Dementia is recognised by WHO (2010) as an international public health priority and by Australia as a national health priority. As a result of the ageing population, the prevalence of dementia is expected to rise exponentially in coming years, with growing economic and emotional costs to society. While a cure for dementia is not yet available, well-being and quality of life can be optimised with adequate care and support services.

A push for community working, and supporting the health and care needs of people within the community rather than within hospital or residential care environments, has highlighted the need for collaboration across sectors, particularly between health and social care, but also housing, law enforcement, etc. The UK policy document *Our Health, Our Care, Our Say* in 2006 emphasised the need for collaboration across these sectors. Similar issues have been highlighted in Australia (Garling, 2008).

What is interprofessional education and how was it developed?

IPE is an overarching term used to describe the theoretical and practical components of an individual's experience. It is defined by the Centre for the Advancement of Interprofessional Education (CAIPE) (2002) as 'those occasions when members (or students) of two or more professions learn with, from and about one another, to improve the collaboration and the quality of care'. The main emphasis, therefore, is the quality of care that an individual or a community receives.

The need for new models of health care for greater collaboration and communication between professionals is most apparent when the breakdown of communication leads to a detrimental effect on a person's health and well-being and, in some cases, premature death.

Collaboration, in the form of communication, is necessary between professionals to ensure quality of care. For IPE to take place, therefore, communication, exchange and collaboration need to take place with, from and about each of the professions in order for it to be called 'interprofessional education'.

Barr (2007) outlines the UK development in IPE between 1966 and 1996, stating that the origins of IPE were often termed 'shared learning', and that these developments were examined earlier by Forman and Nyatanga (1999). Both of these articles outline the need for professions to concentrate on the quality of care of the individual patient, client or community, rather than on the professional background or professional body with which the practitioner may associate. Forman and Nyatanga (1999, 2001) give some insight into why professionals collaborating with each other may find it difficult, by looking at the psychological theory called 'ethnocentricity'. Barr (2007) has outlined the wide variety of work that has taken place since 1966 to improve collaboration between professionals and to break down the barriers, with a view to ensuring the quality of the care of the individual is enhanced, both now and in the future.

Whilst in Australia concerns about collaboration and interprofessional working were not historically highlighted in policy documents (Tope, 1996), some research was undertaken by Owens, Carrier and Horder (1995). It is clear that from mid-2000 onwards both Health Workforce Australia and the Office of Learning and Teaching have been particularly interested in this area and have funded a number of research projects. The first of these was documented by Learning and Teaching for Interprofessional Practice (2009).

Why do we need interprofessional education?

Learning to collaborate

Integrated approach Leutz (1999) defines the integrated approach to care as: 'The search to connect the healthcare system (acute, primary medical and skilled) with other human service systems (e.g. long-term care, education and vocational and housing services) to improve outcomes (clinical, satisfaction and efficiency)'.

International policies and changes in health care delivery call again and again for professionals to learn together and to work together. In its report *Learning Together to Work Together for Health* (1988), WHO called for all regions internationally to consider the benefits of professionals learning together and working together. In 1998, the European region produced a document called *Health for All in the 21st Century*, which incorporated a policy framework colloquially known as 'Health 21'. All UK policies since this time can be linked back to this document and, therefore, to the original WHO policy. Tope (1996) wrote that Health 21:

> is littered with references to the need for collaborative frameworks; **integrated approach**; co-operation; common approaches; pooling of resources; common values; and furthermore

it signals the need to strengthen, adapt and reconfigure models of health service delivery based on evidence of best practice and sustainable strategies.

Meads (2006) found that developed countries, such as Australia, Malaysia, and those in Europe and North America, had similar policies about primary care and, indeed, IPE. Developing countries, such as Algeria, Cameroon, the Dominican Republic, Fiji, the Philippines, Thailand, Sudan, Lebanon, Columbia and South Africa, did not use the terms 'primary care' or 'interprofessional education' but did look at collaborative models and ways of working with a focus on the individual and a much wider context than just health. Meads indicated that India had an excellent example of both primary care and IPE, and that, perhaps, developed countries could still learn from those considered to be developing.

In a report, Health Canada indicated that:

> changing the way we educate health professionals is key to achieving system change and to ensuring that health providers have the necessary knowledge and training to work effectively in interprofessional teams within the evolving health care system. (Hoffman et al., 2008)

In Australia, the Department of Health Western Australia (2006) indicated that universities should develop closer links between medical schools, schools of nursing education and allied health schools, with a view to providing more joint education between health profession students and collectively consider how health professionals should be educated. The report encourages a focus on:

- the patient, individual or community;
- consideration of demographics, human factors, communication and collaboration between members of the health care team;
- quality improvement;
- ethics;
- individual and group care dynamics;
- professional responsibility.

As indicated in Chapter 1, there are many groups internationally that have formed to share good practice in IPE. These include:

- The Network: Towards Unity for Health (The Network: TUFH), which is closely associated with WHO, and has a task force of IPE;
- Canadian Interprofessional Health Collaborative (CIHC);
- Centre for the Advancement of Interprofessional Education (CAIPE), which is UK-based;

- Australasian Interprofessional Practice and Education Network (AIPPEN);
- International Association for Interprofessional Education and Collaborative Practice (InterEd);
- European Interprofessional Practice and Education Network (EIPEN);
- Nordic Interprofessional Network (NIPNET);
- Japan Association for Interprofessional Education (JAIPE);
- American Interprofessional Health Collaborative (AIHC).

In 2014, each of these groups reinforced their agreement to collaborate with each other so that the good practice emerging within each organisation and the networking within each particular group can also be shared internationally. It is interesting to note that, from the early part of this century, The Network: TUFH (a non-governmental organisation in an official relationship with WHO) has worked on the model, concentrating on the delivery of health services based on people's *needs* (at its centre) (see Figure 3.1) in collaboration with policy makers, health professions, academic institutions, communities and health managers.

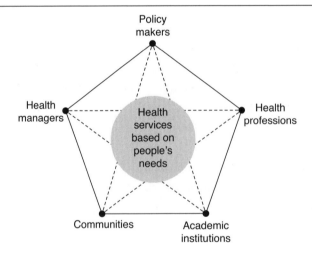

FIGURE 3.1 *The Towards Unity for Health Model (Boelen, 2006) Reproduced with permission from The Network: Towards Unity for Health*

The Towards Unity for Health Model can be effectively used within any country where communities are living in remote locations, whether that is in India or Australia. Academics from universities go out to research what the community actually needs and then individuals from various organisations collaborate to provide for those needs, rather than believing that they already have the answers and implementing processes that fall short of what the community actually requires (Boelen et al., 2007). This model has also been used to show the different IPE networks (see Figure 3.2).

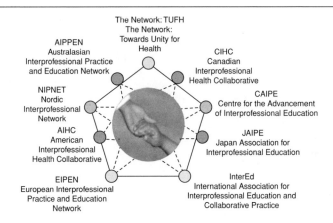

FIGURE
3.2

The Towards Unity for Health pentagon and interprofessional networks (Forman, 2005)

Creating a health workforce for the future

In 2013, WHO reiterated the critical shortage of the health care workforce. The report (Campbell et al., 2013) stated 'the world will be short of 12.9 million health-care workers by 2035; today, 2013, that figure stands at 7.2 million.' The change in demographics of the population internationally, with a higher ageing population and a reducing younger population, means that there will be more health needs for the elderly and fewer people able to go into the professional groups from the younger end.

In 2010, WHO conducted a review of interprofessional practice internationally: the resulting framework is shown in Figure 3.3.

This framework encourages policy makers, health care managers, health care educators and health care teams to study carefully the local population's health care needs and design health care systems for both now and the future. It also ensures that IPE and practice are incorporated into the design so that health care workers can communicate and collaborate together, thereby optimising and strengthening the health care system and improving the health outcomes of the population.

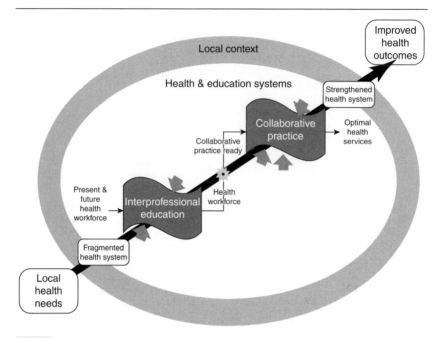

FIGURE 3.3 *The World Health Organization (2010) Framework for Action on Interprofessional Education and Collaborative Practice (WHO, 2010) Reproduced with permission from the World Health Organization.*

As highlighted by Health Workforce Australia (2012), this means that the current models of health care in Australia need to adapt to mitigate the expected increase in health care needs with reduced numbers of staff. The health care professionals need to modify their skills and ways of working to cater for the increase in the older population and their associated health care needs. With fewer in the health care workforce, the communication between them and with the individual needing care is all the more important.

The Australian context for interprofessional education and collaborative practice

Public health services in Australia are implementing unprecedented levels of health service reconfiguration and reform to address the increasing demand and pressure on the system caused by a growing and ageing population, an increase in chronic disease, workforce shortages and the burgeoning cost of health care delivery (Government of Western Australia and Department of Health Western Australia, 2009). With the WHO framework (2010), the changes in health workforce configurations and known changes in demography, it was felt important that Australia undertook a review of how IPE was being implemented and to see if models could be derived to help educators design an interprofessional curriculum.

Four research projects in this area have been funded and the reports on these can be found as follows:

1   Interprofessional Health Education in Australia: The Way Forward (Learning and Teaching for Interprofessional Practice, 2009): http://www. aippen.net/docs/LTIPP_proposal_apr09.pdf

2   Interprofessional Education: A National Audit, 2013 (The Interprofessional Curriculum Renewal Consortium, Australia, 2013): http:// www.hwa.gov.au/sites/.../IPE%20Audit%20report%20Jan%202013. pdf

3   Interprofessional Education for Health Professionals in Western Australia: Perspectives and Activity (Nicol, 2012): http://www.health.wa.gov. au/wactn/.../IPE_For_Health_Professionals_in_WA

4   Curriculum Renewal for Interprofessional Education in Health (The Interprofessional Curriculum Renewal Consortium, Australia, 2014): http://caipe.org.uk/silo/files/ipecurriculum-renewal-20141.pdf

As a result of these projects a four-dimensional interprofessional framework was developed as shown in Figure 3.4.

In using this framework, educators are encouraged to consider carefully four aspects in developing an interprofessional curriculum.

Identifying the future health care practice needs

This dimension invites us to consider carefully the workforce of the future and how we can best educate them to deliver the care needed for the individual or community with which they are working. For example, we may need to reflect on the team of people who will be needed to work with individuals who have

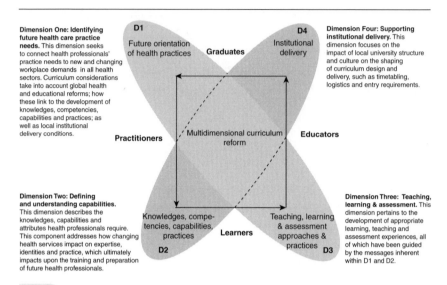

Dimension One: Identifying future health care practice needs. This dimension seeks to connect health professionals' practice needs to new and changing workplace demands in all health sectors. Curriculum considerations take into account global health and educational reforms; how these link to the development of knowledges, competencies, capabilities and practices; as well as local institutional delivery conditions.

D1 Future orientation of health practices   Graduates

D4 Institutional delivery

Dimension Four: Supporting institutional delivery. This dimension focuses on the impact of local university structure and culture on the shaping of curriculum design and delivery, such as timetabling, logistics and entry requirements.

Practitioners   Multidimensional curriculum reform   Educators

Dimension Two: Defining and understanding capabilities. This dimension describes the knowledges, capabilities and attributes health professionals require. This component addresses how changing health services impact on expertise, identities and practice, which ultimately impacts upon the training and preparation of future health professionals.

Knowledges, competencies, capabilities, practices   Learners
D2

Teaching, learning & assessment approaches & practices   D3

Dimension Three: Teaching, learning & assessment. This dimension pertains to the development of appropriate learning, teaching and assessment experiences, all of which have been guided by the messages inherent within D1 and D2.

FIGURE 3.4

The Four-Dimensional Curriculum Development Framework (Lee et al., 2013)
Reproduced with the kind permission of Australian and New Zealand Association of Health Professional Educators Inc.

dementia. Who are the best people to work with these individuals? What sort of mix of skills do we need in this team and how are we going to both encourage and ensure that they will collaborate effectively together with a focus on the needs of the person in their care?

Defining and understanding capabilities

In designing an interprofessional curriculum, we need to consider carefully the capabilities or competencies future health care professionals will need (Nicol & Forman, 2014).

There has recently been a research project undertaken in Australia to develop a work-based assessment tool for interprofessional professional practice (The iTOFT Consortium, Australia, 2015). Along with outlining how interprofessional competencies have been developed, which is reported in Thistlethwaite et al. (2014), the report includes an assessment tool to use in both developing and assessing interprofessional skills. This report will be of value for educators in aligning their teaching and assessment of IPE.

Teaching, learning and assessment

All aspects of teaching, learning and assessment should be considered and aligned in this dimension. The teaching in the classroom, how this is best delivered, the work in skills labs and placements, online learning and self-directed learning, to name but a few, all need to be aligned to ensure that the student gains the knowledge, skills and capabilities needed for working effectively in an interprofessional team. Further consideration of this is given in Cartwright et al. (2013).

Supporting institutional delivery

This dimension ensures that we consider how the curriculum being developed fits with existing systems and processes both within the university and in the practice setting. Are we maximising the resources available to us? Do other resources need to be put in place? Is the correct leadership in place? (Forman, Jones & Thistlethwaite, 2014; Forman, Jones & Thistlethwaite, 2015).

An outline of the research undertaken, with further information on the four projects and guidance on how the model can be used in practice, can be found in Steketee et al. (2014).

The breadth of the health care reform program presents many challenges for those involved in direct patient care, and the management and delivery of health services across all aspects of care. There has been a system focus on health service and infrastructure planning, and the articulation of new interprofessional models of care that will deliver the goals of ensuring a sustainable, safe health service with care closer to home, timely access and improved health outcomes.

It is, therefore, widely accepted that there are many pressures on aged care services throughout the world, driven by the changing needs of the clients, the need to prepare health workers for new roles and new regulatory requirements. The specific needs of clients with dementia due to the ageing population are a key priority.

Conclusion

This chapter provides an insight into the history and development of IPE, its context in health professional education both now and in the future, and why, in the care of the elderly, interprofessional practice is so crucial.

Later chapters will outline the developments taking place in interprofessional dementia care, providing case study examples that look at IPE and practice that will be required for clients with dementia in the future.

Self-directed learning activities

1 There are a variety of health professionals within a health care team. How much do you know about the role of each of the professions in the delivery of health care?

2 Now consider a young person who has dementia. How many health care professionals do you think have seen this person in a week, and how have these professionals communicated their findings to both the young person and the other health care practitioners?

3 If you were designing a health care service for clients with dementia, how would you design a health care model that ensures the needs of the client are the main focus? How would you educate a health care workforce for this health care model?

References

Barr, H. (2007). Interprofessional education: The fourth focus. *Journal of Interprofessional Care*, 21(S2): 40–50. doi: 10.1080/13561820701515335

Boelen, C. (2006). Exemplary network: TUFH field experiences pentagram. *Towards Unity for Health Newsletter*, 25(2). Gent: The Network: Towards Unity for Health.

Boelen, C., Glasser, J., Gofin, J., Lippeveld, T. & Orobaton, N. (2007). Towards unity for health: The quest for evidence. *Education for Health*, 20: 90.

Campbell, J., Dussault, G., Buchan, J., Pozo-Martin, F., Guerra Arias, M., Leone, C., Siyam, A. & Cometto, G. (2013). *A universal truth: No health without a workforce.* Forum Report, Third Global Forum on Human Resources for Health. Recife, Brazil. Geneva: Global Health Workforce Alliance and World Health Organization.

Cartwright, J., Franklin, D., Forman, D. & Freegard, H. (2013). Promoting collaborative dementia care via online interprofessional education. *Australasian Journal of Ageing*. doi: 10.1111/ajag.12106

Centre for the Advancement of Interprofessional Education (CAIPE). (2002). Definition of interprofessional education. Retrieved 30 March 2015 from http://caipe.org.uk/about-us/defining-ipe/

Department of Health Western Australia. (2006). *Educating the present and future health workforce.* Perth: Department of Health Western Australia.

Flexner, A. (1910). Medical education in the United States and Canada: A report to the Carnegie Foundation for the advancement of teaching. New York: The Carnegie Foundation for the Advancement of Teaching.

Forman, D. (2005). Recognising the importance of the interpersonal: The theory–practice relationship in interprofessional education. *Higher Education Academy Health Sciences and Practice,* 7: 55–60.

Forman, D. & Nyatanga, L. (1999). The evolution of shared learning: Some political and professional imperatives. *Medical Teacher,* 21(5): 489–96.

Forman, D. & Nyatanga, L. (2001). The process of developing a research questionnaire to measure attitudes to shared learning. *Medical Teacher,* 23(6): 603–7.

Forman, D., Jones, M. & Thistlethwaite, J. (eds). (2014). *Leadership development for interprofessional education and collaborative practice.* Basingstoke, UK: Palgrave Macmillan.

Forman, D., Jones, M. & Thistlethwaite, J. (eds). (2015). *Leadership and collaboration: Further developments for IPE and collaborative practice.* Basingstoke, UK: Palgrave.

Garling, P. (2008). *Final report of the special commission of inquiry: Acute care in NSW public hospitals, 2008 – Overview.* Retrieved 30 March 2015 from http://www.lawlink.nsw.gov.au/acsinquiry

Government of Western Australia and Department of Health Western Australia. (2009). *WA Health Clinical Services Framework, 2010–2020.* Perth: Department of Health Western Australia.

Health Workforce Australia. (2012). *Doctors, nurses and midwives.* Adelaide: Health Workforce 2025. Retrieved 30 March 2015 from http://www.hwa.gov.au/health-workforce-2025

Hoffman, S.J., Rosenfield, D., Gilbert, J.H.V. & Oandasan, I.F. (2008). Student leadership in interprofessional education: Benefits, challenges and implications for educators, researchers and policymakers. *Medical Education,* 42(7): 654–61.

Learning and Teaching for Interprofessional Practice. (2009). *Interprofessional health education in Australia: The way forward.* Sydney: Learning and Teaching for Interprofessional Practice.

Lee, A., Steketee, C. Rogers, G. & Moran, M. (2013). Towards a theoretical framework for curriculum development in health professional education. *Focus on Health Professional Education: A Multidisciplinary Journal,* 14(3): 64–77.

Meads, G. (2006). Primary health care models: learning across continents. *Primary Health Care Research & Development,* 7(4): 281–3. doi: 10.1017/S1463423606000375

Nicol, P. (2012). *Interprofessional education for health professionals in Western Australia: Perspectives and activity.* Sydney: University of Technology.

Nicol, P. & Forman, D. (2014). Attributes of effective interprofessional placement. *Journal of Research in Interprofessional Practice,* 4(2): 1–11.

Owens, P., Carrier, J. & Horder, J. (1995). *Interprofessional issues in community and primary health care.* London: Macmillan.

Steketee, C., Forman, D., Dunston, R., Yassine, T., Matthews, L.R., Saunders, R., Nicol, P. & Alliex, S. (2014). Interprofessional health education in Australia: Three research projects informing curriculum renewal and development. *Applied Nursing Research*: 27: 115–20.

The Interprofessional Curriculum Renewal Consortium, Australia. (2013). *Interprofessional education: A national audit.* Report to Health Workforce Australia. Sydney: Centre for Research in Learning and Change, University of Technology.

The Interprofessional Curriculum Renewal Consortium, Australia. (2014). *Curriculum Renewal for Interprofessional Education in Health.* Canberra: Commonwealth of Australia, Office of Learning and Teaching.

The iTOFT Consortium, Australia. (2015). *Work based assessment of teamwork: An interprofessional approach.* Canberra: Commonwealth of Australia, Office of Learning and Teaching.

The King's Fund. (2011). *The future of leadership and management in the NHS. No more heroes.* Report from The King's Fund Commission on Leadership and Management in the NHS. London: The King's Fund.

Thistlethwaite, J., Forman, D., Matthews, L., Rogers, G., Steketee, C. & Yassine, T. (2014). Interprofessional education competencies and frameworks in health: A comparative analysis. *Academic Medicine.* June 89(6): 1–7.

Tope, T. (1996). *Integrated interdisciplinary learning between health and social care professions: A feasibility study.* Aldershot: Avebury.

West, B.J., Patera, J.L. & Carsten, M.K. (2009). Team level positivity: Investigating positive psychological capacities and team level outcomes. *Journal of Organisational Behaviour,* 30: 249–67.

World Health Organization (WHO). (1978). *Guidelines for evaluating a training programme for health personnel.* Geneva: WHO.

World Health Organization (WHO). (1988). *Learning together to work together for health: The team approach.* Technical Report Series No. 769. Geneva: WHO.

World Health Organization (WHO). (1998). *Health for all in the 21st century.* European Health for All Series No. 5. Geneva: WHO.

World Health Organization (WHO). (2010). *Framework for action on interprofessional education and collaborative practice.* Retrieved 30 March 2015 from www.who.int/hrh/resources/framework_ction/en/

4 Evidence-based practice

Sue Fyfe, Lyn Phillipson and Michael Annear

Learning outcomes

1 Identify the challenges of applying evidence-based practice to health workplaces.

2 Discuss the role of interprofessional education in supporting the translation of evidence into practice within dementia care.

3 Describe the barriers and enablers of knowledge translation and evidence-based practice.

Key terms

- evaluation

- evidence-based practice (EBP)

- interprofessional education (IPE)

- knowledge translation (KT)

- power

Introduction

The concept of **evidence-based practice (EBP)** has become the gold standard for health care as it envisions that new and innovative findings (ideas, treatments, technology and methods) will be incorporated into the education of health care teams and thus will lead to improvements in real-world practice with the application of current knowledge. It makes sense that we look to the research literature (peer reviewed and published studies), evaluate what we find, and use evidence in our planning and our ways of doing things. The Oxford Centre for Evidence-Based Medicine (Howick et al., 2011) has developed a hierarchy of likely best evidence with five levels of evidence from strongest to weakest: systematic reviews, randomised controlled trials, cohort studies, case series and clinical/mechanistic reasoning. They link the evidence

> **Evidence-based practice (EBP)** Health care professionals who perform evidence-based practice use research evidence along with clinical expertise and patient preferences.

to whether it is being used for diagnosis, prognosis, therapy and prevention, or economic decision analysis. Eccles and colleagues (1998) used three evidence categories to develop guidelines for the primary care management of dementia: They are:

I well-designed randomised controlled trials, meta-analyses or systematic reviews;

II well-designed cohort or case control studies;

III uncontrolled studies or external consensus.

They also use a measure of strength of recommendation based on these three categories:

- directly based on category I evidence;
- directly based on category II evidence;
- directly based on category III evidence OR extrapolated recommendations from category I and II evidence;
- based on clinical opinion from a group.

> **Interprofessional education (IPE)**
>
> Interprofessional education occurs when two or more professions learn with, from and about each other to improve collaboration and the quality of care (http://www.caipe.org.uk/about-us/defining-ipe/). When students from two or more professions learn about, from and with each other to enable effective collaboration and improve health outcomes (WHO, 2010).

But, in practice, do we use evidence to make our decisions, whether it is about the management of dementia, or our view of the world? Our contention is that, while evidence and innovative knowledge should inform practice, it must first be created and then transferred within health care and education systems. This is the state of current work in **interprofessional education (IPE)**.

Challenges of knowledge translation: Applying evidence to practice

Aristotle, in the 4th century BC, determined that the sun moved around the earth (an earth-centric view). It made sense, fitted the observed movements of the star, and the weight of his opinion meant that an early heliocentric ('sun-centred') system, proposed by Aristarchus of Greece (Heath, 2013; Zellik, 2002), did not last long. In the 15th century, Copernicus developed a model with the earth moving around the sun rather than the other way around and later Galileo, using a simple telescope, provided evidence of a sun-centred model, but the evidence did not outweigh dogma and was disbelieved or ignored. Copernicus did not publish his works until near death, thus avoiding the issue (Somervill, 2005). Galileo published *Dialogue*, in which he compared the Aristotelian (earth-centric) and Copernican (sun-centred) views. As a result he faced the Inquisition, was placed under house arrest and refused the rights to have visitors or publish his works (Finocchiaro, 2010). It was not until 1744, 102 years after his death, that the Church lifted its ban on the publication of Galileo's *Dialogue*. Challenging accepted dogma can be very difficult.

In health, Semmelweis, a Hungarian physician, in the 1840s, clearly showed that hand washing greatly reduced post-delivery mortality in the Vienna General Hospital. However, despite showing clear evidence in support of his approach, and convincing some junior doctors of its value, he failed to convince senior staff, who had a different view that improved ventilation had reduced mortality, and did not publish his findings. He was hounded from his post, later suffered a mental breakdown and died in an asylum (Best & Neuhauser, 2004).

The resistance to the introduction of better ways of practice continues, although perhaps without the drastic consequences experienced by Semmelweis. Why does resistance continue in the face of evidence to the contrary? Why do we continue to believe something and act on it when we have good evidence about a better way? To change and counter a prevailing view takes courage when the view is held by powerful forces. Why was Semmelweis ignored? He was ignored because his ideas did not fit into existing views of how the known world was structured, or about the causation of disease before the germ theory (Best & Neuhauser, 2004). The paradigm shift, or scientific revolution, that was needed to accept Semmelweis' view, including the crisis where serious anomalies cannot be reconciled within the existing world view, had not yet occurred (Kuhn, 2012).

Both Galileo and Semmelweis were unable to change the culture of the Church or hospital despite convincing some of the value of their ideas. Those in authority maintained the orthodoxy and protected their professional reputations and positions. Neither was able to develop an environment that was willing to accept new ideas (Best & Neuhauser, 2004). The balance between healthy scepticism of the new and rigid acceptance of the status quo can be difficult to find.

There is currently no lack of evidence or guidelines to inform practice in caring for those with dementia. Guidelines for diagnosis, for treatment and for psychosocial approaches to care and treatment are clear in the literature. Eccles and colleagues (1998) developed evidence-based guidelines for the treatment of dementia using categories of evidence and evaluating strength of recommendations. They had GPs in mind when they developed guidelines, both to help manage patients with dementia and also to help their carers. Throughout the guidelines, published in the *British Medical Journal*, they identify the level of evidence for their statements and recommendations. They identify physical and cognitive screening, risk factors for other conditions, such as falls and depression, and the need for residential care as well as drug therapies available at the time. By 2013, the article had been cited 44 times, indicating that it has had an impact on other researchers; but have they changed practice? The literature also raises concerns about these guidelines not being used (Drake et al., 2001) and it is unknown whether they have resulted in a corresponding change in practice.

The Cochrane Collaboration (2014) provided reviews that helped doctors, patients, policy makers and others make decisions about health care. By April 2014, the Dementia and Cognitive Improvement Group had published 270 reviews on dementia, including 19 on diagnosis and 194 on dementia and chronic cognitive impairment. The Diagnostic and Statistical Manual of Mental Disorders (American Psychiatric Association, 2013) has synthesised evidence and recommendations, and this has resulted in a much revised set of recommendations. However, while evidence is there, it may be inconclusive in some cases (Lyketsos et al., 2006; Köpke & McCleery, 2015) and thus go unrecognised or ignored. (Zipoli & Kennedy, 2005) found that, amongst speech pathologists, clinical experience and colleague opinion was used more than clinical practice guidelines or research studies even when there was a positive response to EBP.

Why don't health care teams evidence their practice?

Changing practice and implementing new ways of doing things is not easy. Even when a change promises to make service faster and more efficient with better outcomes, making the change requires an investment of time and resources in order to overcome institutional/organisational inertia. Both institutional and personal factors can build barriers (McKenna, Ashton & Keeney, 2004; Solomons & Spross, 2011). Workloads are such that few health care teams have the time or energy to invest in improving practice during their employment hours. While most health professional qualifications require evidence of critical thinking, deductive reasoning, knowledge of research methodologies and engagement with current research literature, once in the workforce these skills may not be well used and may be forgotten. In addition new graduates in particular may not see promoting and leading change as part of their role and developing professional identity.

Institutional barriers to EBP occur within strategic, cultural, technical and structural contexts. At a strategic level, leaders and managers within an organisation may consider EBP as a lower priority and invest resources into other aspects of service. Short-term cost constraints and poor staff retention and recruitment practices can increase workloads, limit access to resources and inhibit changes in practice.

At a cultural level, working in a multidisciplinary team, and convincing other professions of the benefits of change, especially if it requires a change in practice as well, can be a barrier. There may also be a lack of respect for, and suspicion of, research and organisational change. Research is not usually a part of everyday clinical practice and to the uninvolved is seen as an activity far re-moved from the practicalities of the workplace. Interpreting and determining transferability of research findings requires a cultural environment – including managers, professionals and care staff – conducive to questioning current prac-tice and an appreciation of research as a means of answering such questions.

At a technical level, inadequate information systems and poor training in IT can make accessing available resources difficult. For example, information may not be compiled and/or stored in one place, making it difficult, and re-quiring advanced IT skills, to find and collate relevant information. Making a change in practice will most likely require different resources that may be difficult to attain.

In organisations with several service sites, consistency of practice is prized highly. At this structural level, implementing change requires a whole organi-sational approach. Taking a proposal from the long and complicated committee process through to the resource-intensive training and implementation phases is daunting.

How can health workers be supported to use evidence in their practice?

How do we most effectively translate new advancements in knowledge and technology into the everyday practices of health workers? While the transfer of quality research into clinical settings is the foundation of EBP, a significant research–practice gap exists. This affects the ease, speed and effectiveness with which new findings are adopted in the care of people with dementia (Davis et al., 2003; Draper et al., 2009). In the past, this process has been viewed as being pushed by researchers as a one-way communication from researcher or educator to practitioners. However, more recently, there has been a growing emphasis on **knowledge translation (KT)**, with the benefits of promoting knowledge exchange between researchers, educators and practitioners, and an emerging view that this can be interactive and mutually advantageous (Mitton et al., 2007). Such principles appear consistent with many of those within the literature on IPE – sharing an emphasis on facilitating the collaboration of health care teams (professionals and care workers) and educators from different backgrounds for the purposes of improving quality of care (Centre for the Advancement of Interprofessional Education, 2002).

> **Knowledge translation (KT)** Knowledge translation is the term often used to describe integration of research into practice where the intent is clear from the beginning of the research (Johnson, 2005).

KT is the term often used to describe integration of research into practice where the intent is clear from the beginning of the research. Johnson (2005) has conceptualised knowledge translation as:

> an active, *multi directional* flow of information which begins at project inception … with interactions that occur before, during and after a project with the goals of developing research questions, setting a research agenda and then determining actions.

Other definitions also acknowledge the complex interaction and exchange that contributes to KT (Davis et al., 2003; Draper et al., 2009). Action research methodology responds to this complexity with its focus on collaboration between researcher and the people in the situation, involving critical enquiry and reflective learning (Checkland & Holwell, 1998). Within this framework, it is clear that the research is intended to change the organisation or system in which the research takes place by empowering and educating workers. However, this ideal and complex interaction between researcher and the situation or organisation does not always take place, and there can be a disconnection between research and practice; this is the research–practice gap that can reduce the effectiveness of KT.

Can education support knowledge translation and reduce this research–practice gap?

Education can be a key with KT seen as an essential 'third stream', linking researchers (universities) and practitioners (industry), and providing continued education for professionals, and thereby reducing the research–practice gap (Phillips, 2006). The conceptualisation of this educational dimension can link research, education and practice with mutual benefit. For example, during 2011–13, the Australian Dementia Training and Study Centre (DTSC) developed and adopted a conceptual framework for 'knowledge transfer and translation' for use within the DTSC education and training programs nationally (Phillipson, Reis & Fleming, 2013) (known as the DTSC KT National Framework). This conceptual framework adapted the work of Phillips (2006) and defined 'knowledge' broadly to be inclusive of information, attitudes (mindsets/cultures), skill, work practices, technologies and other capabilities, relevant to the practices of health care teams in the care of people with dementia. In this context, Phillipson, Reis & Fleming (2013) defined knowledge transfer and KT in this framework to comprise:

> The process of engaging with [undergraduate and graduate] health professionals (and/or their representative employers, professional associations, or tertiary institutions involved in their training) to generate, produce, acquire, apply or make accessible the 'knowledge' (information, skills, capabilities, technologies or other) required to improve the 'the quality of care and support provided to people with dementia and their caregivers'.

They also suggested that, within this framework, effective educational practice to promote KT requires activities to support health care teams in the following domains:

- the identification of knowledge or evidence (knowledge generation);
- the use of high quality educational products, resources and tools (knowledge products);
- the provision of timely access to, and effective dissemination of, evidence (knowledge access);
- support to build, and practise, skills and capacity (knowledge capacity);
- support to build professional relationships to achieve KT outcomes (knowledge relationships).

How knowledge translation affects day-to-day practices of health care teams and educators

As pointed out by Mitton et al. (2007), there is limited evidence evaluating KT and the strategies that actually work in practice. In this light, the DTSC KT National Framework has also adapted the four stage 'Awareness to Adherence'

KT Evaluation Model (known as 'the Pathman Model) (Pathman et al., 1996; Phillipson, Reis & Fleming, 2013). The DTSC KT National Framework defines domains of educational activity that can move students and practitioners from personal awareness through to agreement and adoption, but also extends the Pathman Model to consider the strategies that may be needed to support adherence (sustained practice change) at both a personal and organisational level. In a clinical context, this process of change may be measured by assessing *awareness* using statements such as 'this educational activity (e.g. workshop or lecture) increased my awareness of new knowledge in the area' to *agreement*, such as 'I feel my capacity to address this issue in my workplace has been enhanced by ... the workshop' and 'I agree it is important to change my practice' and 'I intend to try and make a change' then to *adoption* 'I have tried to change my own practice/practice in my workplace as a result of this workshop.' *Adherence* is the final stage, where the DTSC KT National Framework suggests that EBP has been achieved when the new practice becomes 'the way we do things around here'.

These stages of KT **evaluation** relate to many others within the behaviour-change literature, such as those outlined by Procheska and Velicer (1997) in the transtheoretical model of health behaviour change. They proposed that the process of behaviour change involves five stages: pre-contemplation, contemplation, preparation for action, action and maintenance. During this process, initially a person may be aware of a problem or indeed may not, and has no thought of changing their behaviour. When they move to contemplation, they do want to change their behaviour. However, they may not actually do so until they prepare for it and then begin to undertake the new behaviour in the action phase. Once the behaviour has become habitual and undertaken for at least six months, the person enters the maintenance phase. While not specifically aligned with the DTSC KT National Framework, there are clear links between contemplation and awareness, preparation and agreement, action and adoption, and maintenance and adherence. Likewise, there is a motivational aspect to behaviour change that is identified in the health action process approach (Schwarzer, 1992). This approach brings motivation for change into the Pathman Model between awareness and action or adoption. At an organisational level, there are parallels, with resistance to change, especially where innovation is a factor, being an important issue. Lewin (1951) developed the Force Field Analysis Model, where those forces driving changes are resisted by restraining forces. Individuals resist change for many reasons, including a lack of perceived benefit,

Evaluation
Appraisal or value
of something.

fear of failure, sense of threat to existing status and **power**, and dependence (Martin, 2005). Kotter and Schlesinger (2008) identified a number of strategies to help deal with resistance, including education and communication, participation and involvement, and facilitation and support. These strategies respond to individuals and their process of behaviour change.

> **Power** Power, it has been argued, is the ability or capacity to act or to exercise influence. As such, it has many dimensions (gender, race, class, knowledge, etc.) that can impact on interprofessional relations (Baker et al., 2011).

The challenges in supporting EBP in the everyday work practices of students and health care teams, who provide care for people with dementia, are numerous (Draper et al., 2009). Currently, there are few documented cases of 'best practice' strategies providing examples of the types of activities that can be effective in supporting practitioners and students to move through the steps from awareness and agreement, through to adoption and adherence. In the absence of any recognised evidence-based guidelines for training that supports this process, the DTSC KT National Framework has provided educational exemplars of KT that are being utilised to support health care teams to move through these steps (Phillipson, Reis & Fleming, 2013). These exemplars provide cases of leadership in dementia education with the aim of countering existing barriers to change, such as unmet learning needs, silos within the health sector and missed opportunities to involve learners in the provision of care for people with dementia (with appropriate supervision). They can provide students and practitioners with examples of components that are being utilised within the DTSC KT National Framework to support KT (the transition from awareness to agreement and adoption and adherence). They also lead through to the building of relationships and organisational capacity that can support adherence to EBP in dementia care through the engagement of both undergraduate and graduate health professionals.

KT from the VIC–TAS DTSC: The Teaching Residential Aged Care Facility Program (TACFP)

Case study

Within the DTSC KT National Framework exemplars, there is a case that applies IPE to support KT (Phillipson, Reis & Fleming, 2013). This exemplar, conducted within Tasmania, represents a program of action-oriented research (beginning in 2011) to develop a network of teaching aged care facilities (analogous with teaching nursing homes in the US). The aim of the program is to improve student knowledge (knowledge awareness) of dementia palliative care, respond to projected workforce needs in residential aged care, improve organisational culture and capacity (knowledge capacity), and provide students with a positive and collaborative experience of working with peers from the disciplines of nursing medicine and paramedicine (knowledge relationships). The research also supports KT through collaborations (knowledge relationships) among university academics (researchers and tutors), aged care staff (mentors and senior managers) and student learners (Robinson et al., 2013). These collaborations support the transfer of knowledge about best-practice care, treatment and management at the research–practice nexus.

One of the mechanisms for achieving KT in this context is through the vehicle of IPE. IPE is a critical activity for raising 'awareness' about EBP, and providing pathways to agreement with and adoption of strategies that change behaviours (knowledge capacity), and have meaningful health outcomes for residents with dementia and other conditions.

An integral focus on EBP, within these interprofessional clinical placements in residential aged care facilities (RACFs), is made through student assessment of residents, reviews of health histories and current medication regimens, formal presentation of recommendations to facility staff, and implementation and tracking of recommendations over time. These activities are woven into an overarching IPE component of the placement. As many of the students are in their penultimate year of study (for example, fifth year medical students and second year fast-track nursing students), they have a high level of knowledge about current best practice guidelines in the assessment, management and treatment of a range of conditions that affect older people in RACFs. In this sense, the IPE activity provides an avenue for modelling best practice to both peers (student learners from other disciplines) and facility staff in ways that support awareness, agreement, adoption and adherence to the most appropriate strategies for care and treatment.

Two Hobart-based RACFs routinely host students from the University of Tasmania within the context of a teaching aged care facility development program. The length of placement for student groups varies by discipline. Nursing students undertake an embedded clinical placement for two–four weeks, while medical and paramedic students participate for one week. Placements run during defined periods throughout the year and over 1 000 students have completed clinical placements within the program to date. Student group placements are scheduled to ensure that they coincide with their interdisciplinary peers, and in most instances this results in the deliberate alignment of second year nursing students with either fifth year medical students or second year paramedic students.

At the beginning of the placement, all interprofessional students are given an introductory information session, by a tutor, about the importance of interprofessional engagement and what is meant by 'interprofessional ways of working'. Students are also introduced to their interprofessional team members and their allocated resident. Over the course of the week-long engagement, each student works interprofessionally to assess the health and quality of life of one resident, usually with a focus on a particular health issue such as falls, wandering, depression, cultural needs and other concerns that are relevant to their current quality of life. The assessment process challenges students in a number of ways, as all residents selected have a cognitive impairment (usually dementia) and multiple comorbidities. The process of collaborative assessment of a cognitively impaired resident forces students to work together and draw on all of their interpersonal communication and clinical/diagnostic skills. Moreover, the assessment process also challenges facility staff who must address students' queries about the rationale for current treatment approaches.

Over the course of the week, students spend approximately 12 hours interacting with their resident and IPE partner/s. Students assess residents for up to 1.5 hours using tools specific to their disciplines. For example, nursing students may undertake a falls assessment, medical students may undertake a comprehensive medical assessment, and paramedic students may assess a resident's pain. Students then prepare a 10-minute presentation that considers the resident's bio-psycho-social background, identifies a current health issue that is not managed optimally or which is causing problems for the resident, and make evidence-based recommendations for clinical staff. At the end of the presentations, students provide a copy to the mentor leader and include a summary of their recommendations in the resident's file as a reference for the resident's GP. Following the assessments and presentations to facility staff, the mentor leader (usually a senior registered nurse within the facility) collects student recommendations, sets up a process for implementing those that are most appropriate and tracks the outcomes.

This process is assigned to a particular staff member, who is responsible for their implementation and tracking by a series of follow-up assessments at four, eight and 12 weeks, following the completion of the IPE exercise. Knowledge products developed from the IPE activity include a protocol for collaborative assessment between interdisciplinary groups, recorded student recommendations for improvements in resident care, and an implementation and outcomes log for staff to track the effectiveness of student-initiated changes in care.

The IPE activity simulates health professional interaction for students in a supervised, yet challenging, clinical setting. Knowledge outcomes, expressed by students as a result of the interprofessional interaction, include a deeper understanding of the role of their peers, opportunities to learn about different assessment techniques, understanding alternative communication strategies with people who have cognitive disorders, opportunities to problem solve and act in a more autonomous fashion (setting them up for forthcoming internship experiences) and modelling EBP for their interdisciplinary partners and mentors. The IPE activity not only helps students to improve their knowledge of dementia, assessment skills and interpersonal communication, but it also builds capacity among the RACF staff (the mentor group) by challenging potentially outmoded knowledge and providing an audit of current resident management. This is achieved through student questioning of the rationale for specific approaches to care and treatment, expectations by facility management for all staff to engage in the teaching of students, the formal assessment/auditing of resident care plans and medication regimens, and expectations for staff to respond to identified deficiencies in resident care raised through the IPE process. This, in turn, supports the organisational change component of the TACFP by adding value for clinical staff, forcing them to reflect on how their knowledge and practice aligns (or does not align) with current best practice and to adhere to a process of continuous improvement.

(Reproduced with permission from the DTSC)

The interprofessional education exemplar and the DTSC KT National Framework

Through the lens of the DTSC KT National Framework, the KT activities of the TACFP exemplar were focused on helping to build the capacity of both students and practitioners for EBP in dementia care, leading to an emphasis on strategies that would raise both knowledge awareness, and address attitudes (agreement) and practice behaviours (adoption and adherence).

This first occurred through the creation of 'knowledge products'. Within this exemplar, they included a structured palliation curriculum for aged care placements focusing on dementia and the complex presentations in aged care, a protocol document explaining and directing the IPE activity, a formalised process for implementing and tracking student recommendations for improvements in resident care, and a protocol document for the development of teaching aged care facilities in Australia. 'Knowledge tools' were also developed to support organisational change. Examples of specific tools include a suite of resources 'Developing and testing a strategy to enhance a palliative approach and care continuity for people with severe and end stage dementia' developed from a 2010–11 research project at Curtin University, WA, and the University of Tasmania (Toye et al., 2012).

'Knowledge access' and 'knowledge relationships' were facilitated within this case study by drawing upon an established research relationship with a prototype teaching aged care facility established 10 years before the inception of the student placement and IPE processes. Within this facility, up to 20 mentors supported the student placement and IPE endeavours, and all staff were given the role of supporting learning, and aligning their practice and professional development with the organisation's goals of becoming a teaching aged care facility. As such, existing 'knowledge relationships' promoted successful participation in the program.

In Tasmania, student placements now continue, with formal commitments from both the University of Tasmania and participating RACFs (recognised in memoranda of understanding and formal funding arrangements to support the work of a mentor leader based at each facility). Adherence to the Teaching Aged Care Facility Program and IPE activity recognises the multi-faceted benefits for student learning and staff professional development.

As shown in the Tasmanian IPE case study, the most important element of developing sustainable KT partnerships (knowledge relationships) is often the provision of evidence of useful, appropriate outcomes for industry partners. Evidence of improvement in staff knowledge (knowledge awareness) and health/quality of life benefits for residents are a powerful incentive for sustaining such programs. The case study also noted the need for strategic knowledge relationships, not just with the participating aged care facilities, but also with residents and families. This demonstrates the integral use of knowledge relationships within IPE as a mechanism for supporting knowledge capacity.

The IPE case study clearly demonstrates the importance of approaches that engage not just students but also professionals in their workplaces, in a process of change. This case study shows that IPE placements and mentor/mentee relationships (knowledge relationships) between the two RACFs involved provide a structure that increases the chance for staff to be more receptive of changes in behaviour or policy. This in turn prompts greater awareness of the 'evidence' both gained and required. Within the case study, the IPE approach included strategies to increase the support for practice change within RACFs. In particular it provided intensive active support of comprehensive organisational design review and supported the establishment of 'learning and teaching' environments through the structure of the IPE placements.

Enablers of KT and EBP

Enablers of KT, and thus EBP, were embedded in the model and approach of the IPE case study. Enablers included working with the whole RACF and tailoring programs to meet its needs, engaging management and executives in the process of facilitating change, using the capacity for the DTSC to build trust and respect within organisations, ensuring the delivery of support not just training, and working with an organisation that was already engaged in a change process.

Barriers to KT and EBP

Barriers to KT and EBP were mainly identified in the organisational context, and included insufficient time and funding to undertake or sustain projects.

Engaging RACFs in data collection, as part of their core business, was also a barrier to evaluating KT outcomes. Data collection was a challenge for the case study in terms of IPE data, as well as resident outcomes information. The prevailing issues were lack of time, lack of research experience (for example, familiarity with ethical requirements), and lack of understanding about how research can drive change and quality improvement. However, these barriers have now been addressed in the case study facility with the employment of an innovation manager and research support staff to facilitate data collection.

Other barriers included negative organisational inertia (resistance to change), staff fears about being challenged in their knowledge or caught out (lacking crucial understanding), lack of understanding among some academic partners about the value of IPE, lack of research experience among RACF partners (threatening evaluation processes), lack of reliable RACF mentor support in some cases (staff absence and rotation of mentor group membership/leadership), and students sometimes seen as an unwanted imposition on facilities.

Note: The DTSCs are funded by the Australian Government Department of Social Services. Visit www.dss.gov.au for more information.

Conclusion

This exemplar of IPE from within the DTSC program in Victoria and Tasmania provides an example of how IPE can support students and practitioners to promote KT and ultimately EBP. The IPE case study not only highlights the importance of supporting students through a process that moves them from 'awareness' through to 'agreement', but also highlights the important role that IPE can play as an approach to supporting the building of 'knowledge relationships' and the creation of environments in which 'knowledge capacity' can be built in both individuals and organisations. This is important to support the initial 'adoption' of evidence and the movement towards 'adherence' and to a situation where EBP is 'the way we do things around here'.

Self-directed learning activities

1   Why are randomised controlled trials regarded as providing better evidence for practice than a case control or cohort study?

2 What do you think are the most important barriers to implementing EBP in clinical practice?
3 What are knowledge transfer and KT, and how has the framework they provide been used in the DTSC program?
4 How has the DTSC KT National Framework been used in the training of health professional students in Australia?
5 How does interprofessional practice/education support KT and EBP in a health care setting?

Learning extension

1 If you were working in an aged care facility, how would you assess how well, if at all, EBP was being used to care for and treat the residents?
   a Consider unplanned hospitalisation, resident and family member complaints, aggressive episodes and falls rates.
   b Consider facility policies and procedures, and alignment with national evidence-based best practice guidelines in the management of vulnerable clients.
   c Consider participation in lifestyle and leisure activities that promote activity, inclusion and socialisation.
   d Consider staff professional development and ongoing education.
   e Consider participation in university research, and collaboration with clinicians and academics to audit care quality and outcomes.
2 Consider this situation in an aged care facility: You are a new graduate and you have just been employed in your chosen field in this facility. You are given a number of elderly residents on your case load and you start to review their situation and capacity to engage in activities of daily living. You realise that falls are a major problem for some of these residents but, although they are assessed for falls risk when they enter the aged care facility, there does not seem to be any program to reduce the risk of falling. However, it is not your specific job to assess or intervene. You can see that interprofessional practice would be very useful but you are not sure how to go about this without offending your more senior colleagues.
   a What barriers to implementing a falls assessment regimen are you likely to encounter as a new graduate working in an aged care facility?
   b How might the DTSC KT National Framework be useful?
   c How might you go about advocating for change in this setting?

References

American Psychiatric Association. (2013). *Diagnostic and statistical manual of mental disorders* (5th edn). Arlington, VA: American Psychiatric Association.

Best, M. & Neuhauser, D. (2004). Ignaz Semmelweiss and the birth of infection control. *Quality Safety in Health Care*, 13: 233–4. doi:10.1136/qshc.2004010918

Centre for the Advancement of Interprofessional Education (CAIPE). (2002). Defining IPE. Retrieved 16 February 2015 from http://caipe.org.uk/resources/defining-ipe/

Checkland, P. & Holwell, S. (1998). Action research: Its nature and validity. *Systemic Practice and Action Research*, 11(1): 9–21.

Davis, D., Zwarenstein, M., Perrier, L., Rappolt, S., Jadad, A., Evans, M., & Straus, S. (2003). The case for knowledge translation: Shortening the journey from evidence to effect. *British Medical Journal*, 327(7405): 33–5.

Drake, R.E., Goldman, H.H., Leff, S., Lehman, A.F., Dixon, L., Mueser, K.T. & Torrey, W.C. (2001). Implementing evidence-based practices in routine mental health service settings. *Psychiatric Services*, 52(2): 179–82. doi:10.1176/appi.ps.52.2.179

Draper, B., Low, L.F., Withall, A., Vickland, V. & Ward, T. (2009). Translating dementia research into practice. *International Psychogeriatrics*, 21(S1): S72–S80.

Eccles, M., Clarke, J., Livingstone, M., Freemantle, N. & Mason, J. (1998). North of England evidence-based guidelines development project: Guideline for the primary care management of dementia. *British Medical Journal*, 317(7161): 802–8.

Finocchiaro, M.A. (2010). *Defending Copernicus and Galileo: Critical reasoning in the two affairs*. New York: Springer.

Heath, T. (2013). *Aristarchus of Samos, the ancient Copernicus: A history of Greek astronomy to Aristarchus, together with Aristarchus's treatise on the size and distances of the sun and moon*. New York: Cambridge University Press.

Howick, J., Chalmers, I., Glasziou, P., Greenhalgh, T., Heneghan, C., Liberati, A. … Thornton, H. (2011). *Explanation of the 2011 Oxford Centre for Evidence-Based Medicine (OCEBM) levels of evidence (introductory document)*. Oxford: CEBM.

Johnson, L.S. (2005). From knowledge transfer to knowledge translation: Applying research to practice. *OT Now*, July/August, 11–14.

Köpke, S. & McCleery, J. (2015). *Systematic reviews of case management: Too complex to manage?* Retrieved 14 April 2015 from http://www.cochranelibrary.com/editorial/10.1002/14651858.ED000096

Kotter, J.P. & Schlesinger, L.A. (2008). Choosing strategies for change. *Harvard Business Review*, 86(7/8): 130–139.

Kuhn, T.S. (2012). *The structure of scientific revolutions*. Chicago: University of Chicago Press.

Lewin, K. (1951). *Field theory in social science.* London: Harper Row.

Lyketsos, C.G., Colenda, C.C., Beck, C. & Blank, K. (2006). Position statement of the American Association for Geriatric Psychiatry regarding principles of care for patients with dementia resulting from Alzheimer's disease. *American Journal of Geriatric Psychiatry*, 14(7): 61–73.

Martin, J. (2005). *Organisational behaviour and management* (3rd edn). London: Thompson Learning.

McKenna, H.P., Ashton, S. & Keeney, S. (2004). Barriers to evidence-based practice in primary care. *Journal of Advanced Nursing*, 45(2): 178–89.

Mitton, C., Adair, C.E., McKenzie, E., Patten, S.B. & Perry, B.W. (2007). Knowledge transfer and exchange: Review and synthesis of the literature. *Milbank Quarterly*, 85(4): 729–68.

Pathman, D.E., Konrad, T.R., Freed, G.L., Freeman, V.A. & Koch, G.G. (1996). The awareness-to-adherence model of the steps to clinical guideline compliance. *Medical Care*, 34(9): 873–89.

Phillips, K. (2006). *Knowledge transfer and Australian universities and publicly funded research agencies.* Canberra:Department of Education, Science and Training, Australian Government.

Phillipson, L., Reis, S. & Fleming, R. (2013). *National knowledge transfer research for the dementia training and study centres in Australia.* Wollongong: University of Wollongong.

Procheska, J.O. & Velicer, W.F. (1997). The transtheoretical model of health behavior change. *American Journal of Health Promotion*, 12(1): 38–48.

Robinson, A, Lea, E., Tierney, L., See, C., Marlow, A., Morley, C. ... Eccleston, C. (2013). *Teaching aged care facilities: Implementing interprofessional prevocational education and practice in residential aged care.* Hobart: Wicking Dementia Research and Education Centre, University of Tasmania.

Schwarzer, R. (1992). *Self-efficacy: Thought control of action.* Washington, DC: Hemisphere Publishing Corp.

Solomons, N.M. & Spross, J.A. (2011). Evidence-based practice barriers and facilitators from a continuous quality improvement perspective: An integrative review. *Journal of Nursing Management*, 19(1): 109–20.

Somervill, B. (2005). *Nicolaus Copernicus: Father of modern astronomy.* Minneapolis: Compass Point Books.

The Cochrane Collaboration. (2014). *Interprofessional collaboration: Effects of practice-based interventions on professional practice and healthcare outcomes.* Retrieved 29 April 2014 from http://www.cochrane.org

Toye, C., Robinson, A.L., Jiwa, M., Andrews, S., McInerney, F., Horner, B. ... Stratton, B. (2012). Developing and testing a strategy to enhance a palliative approach and care continuity for people who have dementia: Study overview and protocol. *BMC Palliative Care*, 11(1): 4.

Zellik, M. (2002). *Astronomy: The evolving universe* (9th edn). Cambridge, UK: Cambridge University Press.

Zipoli, R.P. & Kennedy, M. (2005). Evidence-based practice among speech-language pathologists: Attitudes, utilization, and barriers. *American Journal of Speech-language Pathology*, 14(3): 208–20. doi: 10.1044/1058–0360(2005/021)

Leadership in interprofessional dementia care

Dawn Forman and Dimity Pond

Learning outcomes

1   Outline why interprofessional leadership is required.

2   Describe the leadership skills required to facilitate interprofessional practice.

3   Discuss the development of interprofessional leadership within the interprofessional practice context.

Key terms

● capabilities

● dementia

● leadership

Leadership

> Some are born to leadership; some achieve leadership; others have leadership thrust upon them.

> Marie's letter to Malvolio in Shakespeare's *Twelfth Night*

Introduction

Historically health service provision has worked on a hierarchical system of **leadership** in which the doctor has been seen to be the lead both legally and ultimately in practice for any decisions about a patient's care. However, practice is starting to change. In 2000, in Canada, the legislation changed to ensure that any health professional could be nominated as leader and is then legally responsible for the care of the individual.

Why has this move away from doctors always being legally responsible happened? In many situations the doctor is not always

> **Leadership**
> Leadership is a process of social influences that maximise the efforts of others towards the achievement of a goal.

present or reachable, for example, in remote, rural locations and some community settings. As Australia has an increasingly ageing population, there are not enough doctors and other health care professionals to service their needs. This has led to the realisation that new health care models and ways of working need to be developed. Health Workforce Australia (HWA) (2012) stated:

> The projections contained in HW [Health Workforce] 2025 show us that unless we start doing things differently, Australia is going to experience continuing health care shortages. To build a health workforce that is able to meet the health care needs of the Australian community in a sustainable way, the next steps will involve seeking national agreement on the actions identified, progressing outcomes through collaboration and consultation and implementing results across health and higher education sectors.

It is not just Australia where these changes are needed and Australia is not alone in believing that collaboration is key. Oandasan et al. (2006) found that collaboration is likely the key to addressing problems such as staff shortage, work related stress, and burn out in the health workforce.

Over the past decade, numerous interprofessional education and collaborative practice initiatives have taken place internationally. Some were initiated as a result of the World Health Organization's (2010) Framework for Action on Interprofessional Education and Collaborative Practice as outlined in Chapter 3 (see Figure 3.3).

Leadership competencies

HWA (2013) has, therefore, looked at the leadership **capabilities** required for the new leaders working in these collaborative environments and has identified a clear goal: leadership for a people-focused health system that is equitable, effective and sustainable, namely:

Capabilities
Forman, Jones & Thistlethwaite (2014) define capability as 'has been used in preference to competence in one IPE framework, as it is considered by some educators to reflect more optimally the necessity that learners and professionals respond and adapt to health care and systems changes'.

- 'People-focused' aligns with evidence that the best health care has the person at its centre, and that workplace satisfaction leads to better clinical and consumer outcomes.
- 'Health system' includes all the organisations and people whose primary purpose is to improve health.
- 'Equitable' reflects evidence that health inequalities exist within populations, and hospitals and health care services can be sources of inequality for patients, clients and workers.
- 'Effective' means the best possible clinical, consumer, quality and team outcomes.
- 'Sustainable' focuses on meeting the health care needs of both current and future generations.

It also identified five capabilities through a process of consultation and review of international work. In June 2013, these capabilities were approved by the Australian Health Ministers' Advisory Council as a nationally agreed health leadership framework.

Figure 5.1 shows how these identified capabilities work together. The detailed descriptions of these capabilities are given in Table 5.1.

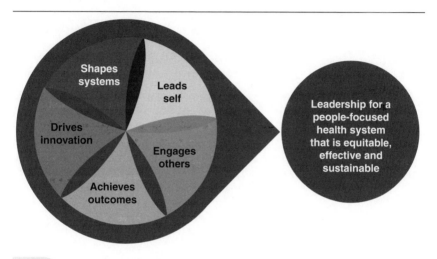

FIGURE
5.1
Leadership capabilities (HWA, 2013)
Reproduced with permission from Health LEADS Australia.

TABLE 5.1 *Leadership capabilities (HWA, 2013)*

LEADS SELF

A leader is always a work in progress. A leader knows their strengths and limitations, and commits to self-reflection and improvement. A leader understands and displays self-awareness, self-regulation, motivation, empathy, and social skills. A leader demonstrates integrity in their role and context, and shows resilience in challenging situations.

CAPABILITIES	DESCRIPTORS
Is self-aware	Understands and manages the impact of their background, assumptions, values and attitudes on themselves and others
Seeks out and takes opportunities for personal development	Actively reflects on their performance as a leader and assumes responsibility for engaging in learning and growth
Has strength of character	Is honest, trustworthy and ethical, and models integrity, courage and resilience

»

ENGAGES OTHERS

A leader enables people to engage with a vision or goal through stories and explanations that make sense of complexity. A leader encourages others to see and accept opportunities to contribute, learn and grow.

CAPABILITIES	DESCRIPTORS
Values diversity and models cultural responsiveness	Recognises first Australians, and ensure that all people, including consumers and workers are treated with dignity and respect in all health care settings
Communicates with honesty and respect	Is approachable, listens well, presents ideas and issues clearly, and participates in difficult conversations with consumers and colleagues with humility and respect
Strengthens consumers, colleagues and others	Inspires and enables others to share ideas and information, to take opportunities to grow and lead, and to collaborate for high performing groups and teams

ACHIEVES OUTCOMES

A leader is a person who works to make a difference. A leader sets a direction that is inspiring and motivating, enables energy and effort to succeed and keeps an eye on the goal. A health leader works with compassion to influence the quality of care and the sustainability of the system.

CAPABILITIES	DESCRIPTORS
Influences and communicates the direction	Collaborates with consumers, colleagues and others to identify, influence and set goals that achieve the vision
Is focused and goal oriented	Influences alignment of resources and decisions with goals and evidence to enable quality, people-centred health work and continuous improvement
Evaluates progress and is accountable for results	Continually monitors and improves, celebrates achievements and holds self and others accountable for individual and service outcomes

DRIVES INNOVATION

Innovation in health is not just for a new product. It includes fundamental changes to business and models of care to achieve people-centred quality services. A key factor for successful innovation is passionate leadership, without which the status quo cannot be challenged.

CAPABILITIES	DESCRIPTORS
Champions the need for innovation and improvement	Inspires and leads others to question, recognise where change is needed, canvas possibilities, support fresh thinking, take risks and collaborate for improvement
Builds support for change	Influences informed discussion on health issues in every encounter, encourages diverse voices and consumer involvement and advocates for better outcomes
Positively contributes to spreading innovative practice	Initiates and maintains momentum for assessing, sharing and celebrating changes for people-centred service and system improvement

SHAPES SYSTEMS

Health is a complex, evolving system where all the parts, including services, legislation and funding, are interconnected. A change in one part has implications for the whole. A leader recognises patterns of interdependency, is able to explain trends, and facilitate strategies that achieve maximum benefits and minimise unintended harm or negative consequences.

》

CAPABILITIES	DESCRIPTORS
Understands and applies systems thinking	Communicates system awareness and negotiates within and across health teams, services and sectors to improve individual and local health outcomes
Engages and partners with consumers and communities	Involves consumers and communities in decision making for health policy, education and training, and health care delivery and improvement
Builds alliances	Promotes understanding, respect and trust between different groups, professions, organisations, sectors and points of view to enable effective collaboration, enhance connectivity, and minimise unintended consequences

Reproduced with permission from Health LEADS Australia.

These leadership capabilities, blended with the interprofessional capabilities that we identified in our MIPPE-D Framework, should help develop our health care workers to work in any environment. The following case study, in a **dementia** care setting, illustrates the changes in leadership that are occurring in this interprofessional environment.

Dementia
Dementia is now referred to as a neurocognitive disorder (NCD) (American Psychiatric Association, 2013), that is, the result of chronic or progressive damage to the brain.

Interprofessional leadership

Case study

Helga Merl, Emily Conway and Dimity Pond, University of Newcastle, Australia

In 2012, funding was made available by the Australian government for projects involving nurse practitioners (NPs) in aged care. In Newcastle, funding was obtained for a collaborative project run by the Discipline of General Practice at the University of Newcastle and the Hunter Medicare Local. Medicare Locals were established by the Australian government in 2011 to work with GPs and other primary health care providers to ensure population access to effective primary health care services (www.yourhealth. gov.au).

The project aimed to employ an NP to assess patients with cognitive difficulties referred by GPs or GP practice nurses. The NP was designated as the 'nurse practitioner mobile memory clinic' (MMC) because she saw patients in their homes.

All names in the case below have been changed to ensure confidentiality.

The Case

Mr Smith was a 76-year-old gentleman referred to the MMC by the practice nurse, Wendy. Wendy had attended a home visit to conduct a routine 75+ Health Assessment and, even though Mr Smith had scored well on the short cognitive screening tool used, she felt things weren't quite right. Mr Smith agreed that he had trouble with his memory. On returning to the surgery, Wendy brought Mr Smith's case to the attention of the GP, Dr Brown, who had agreed to a referral to the MMC and pre-emptively ordered a dementia screen blood pathology battery.

The MMC NP attended a home visit to assess for anxiety, depression, cognition deficits, functional decline, quality of life and behavioural change in Mr Smith, and carer burden, stress, anxiety, depression, coping and quality of life for Mrs Smith. A summary of Mr Smith's results are presented in Table 5.2 Both Mr Smith and his wife had concerns about his memory and word finding difficulties of late. They both described his memory and concentration as poor. He had insight into his memory and language deficits, explaining that he could no longer remember events that he should and no longer enjoyed large family gatherings, as he was embarrassed by word finding difficulties.

TABLE 5.2 *Cognitive screens*

TOOL	DESCRIPTION	RESULT
CCSD	The Cornell Scale for Depression in Dementia (Alexopoulos et al., 1988) is an informant and patient interview to assess signs and symptoms of depression. Scores above 10 indicate a probable major depression.	8/38
GAI-SF	The Geriatric Anxiety Inventory Short Form (Byrne & Pachana, 2011) is a five question screening test providing assessment of anxiety. At cut off scores of three or more, sensitivity is 75% and specificity 87% to anxiety.	5/5
QOL-AD	The Quality of Life in Alzheimer's Disease Scale (Logsdon et al., 2002) is a 13-item measure designed specifically to obtain a rating of the patient's quality of life from both the patient and the caregiver. Total possible score 52.	Patient: 36/52 Informant: 34/52
CAMCOG	The Cambridge Cognitive Examination Revised (Huppert et al., 1995) is a neuropsychological test for the assessment of a range of cognitive functions in elderly people needed to diagnose dementia and to identify mild cognitive impairment. Cut off scores of 80/81 sensitivity is 93% and specificity 87% to dementia.	82/105

Mr Smith had a significant history of head injury with loss of consciousness following a car accident in 1970. Then, 22 years' ago, Mr Smith had a subarachnoid haemorrhage and was in a coma for a number of days. Recently Mr Smith had a prostatectomy. Since this time, both he and his wife had noted worsening of his memory and language problems. He has also lost his sense of humour.

Of relevance was his medical history of long-standing hypertension, depression and melanoma (1998). He had had a recent fall and close falls. He was still driving. His medications were reviewed and anticholinergic antidepressants were noted to be amongst them. He was an ex-smoker, smoking two packets of cigarettes a day for 20 years from age 35 years to 54 years. He was a non-drinker. He had no family history of dementia.

Wendy had suggested a sleep chart to be kept for one week for the NP to review; however, Mr Smith forgot about doing this. Mr and Mrs Smith slept in separate rooms because of his snoring. Mr Smith felt tired through the day. In general he found it difficult to get to sleep, retiring at 9 pm and taking a couple of hours or longer to fall asleep. He got up once to the toilet and went back to sleep easily then and rose around 6 am. On average, he was getting six hours of sleep per night. He was having a nap of late through the day, and the NP discussed sleep hygiene and an appropriate sleep regime.

Physical examination

On examination, Mr Smith's phonation and fluency were normal; he was well dressed. Pulse 54, irregular rhythm with murmur noted on auscultating the heart. BP 170/80 on sitting and standing. Slightly stooped, he had a good gait and arm swing. The sit-to-stand test was normal.

Advance care planning

Mr Smith identified his wife, Marian Smith, as the person responsible and she was involved in a range of legal documentation. No advance care plan (ACP) had been made. The NP discussed nominating someone younger in the family as a backup and making an ACP.

Carer assessment

Overall, Mrs Smith had a good quality of life and was satisfied with her health. Mrs Smith experienced mild burden in her caring role. Mrs Smith used the adaptive coping mechanism of distraction, looking for ways to improve the situation, expressing negative feelings and accepting the reality of the changes in her husband. This helped her manage the impact of her husband's cognitive symptoms on herself.

Interdisciplinary team meeting

A case discussion with the GP and practice nurse was organised. The NP presented the case and the following points were discussed:

> The blood pathology results ordered by the GP were normal.

> Irregular heartbeat and a murmur were discussed. These may also have contributed to memory problems via emboli. The GP agreed to follow up with a Holter monitor.

> The high BP was discussed. It was agreed that this vascular risk factor should be reduced to slow down progression of cognitive impairment. It was unclear if the patient was remembering to take blood pressure medications. A pharmacy Webster- pak was organised.

> Snoring was discussed. It was agreed that sleep apnoea might be a diagnosis, with the GP to follow up on this.

> The use of antidepressants was discussed. It was agreed that anxiety and depression often accompany symptoms of hippocampal involvement causing memory loss and word finding difficulties. However, it was likely that Mr Smith had lived with anxiety and depression for most of his adult life so these were unlikely to be secondary to dementia. It was also likely that they, and the current anticholinergic antidepressants, were impacting on cognition, meaning that it would be worth following this through to see if cognition could be improved through a change in antidepressant treatment. It was

agreed that the GP would do a mental health plan and refer the patient to the Specialist Mental Health Services for Older Persons (SMHSOPs). Medication would be reviewed and a management plan for depressive symptoms and anxiety arranged by the SMHSOPs team (psychogeriatrician and nurse).

> Brain health promotion activities were discussed for reinforcement by the practice nurse when Mr Smith visited the practice. The practice nurse suggested that the local Men's Shed might be a place where he could socialise as well as engage in activities.

At this point, the likely diagnosis was amnestic mild cognitive impairment. Repeat testing at six months was planned.

Second home visit

A follow-up home visit was organised. A management plan for brain health and advanced care planning was attended.

Mr Smith agreed to the following brain health and general management activities:

1 exercise: bodywork through the local HeartMoves program;

2 diet and medications: adding more brightly coloured fruits and vegetables (antioxidants) to an already good diet. Adding over-the-counter Omega 3 supplements as he was eating fish only once a week. Good management of health conditions in partnership with Dr Brown and Wendy. A Webster pak from the pharmacist;

3 cognition: regular monitoring of his BP brain exercises: Mr Smith found that he is not able to concentrate on traditional activities such as crosswords. He will instead brush his hair and teeth and do tasks a few times a day with the opposite hand to normal – his left hand;

4 fun: working in his shed, which he did often. He agreed to try the Men's Shed although he found talking to men distracted him from his work! He found travelling fun so he and Mrs Smith agreed to go on more weekend trips;

5 noisy and crowded situations: Mr Smith was told to always have a quiet room available to manage his inability to screen out competing stimuli and assist cognition. He should also let his family know that he will find one-on-one, rather than group, interaction enjoyable;

6 sleep: Mr Smith was happy to have an afternoon nap to recharge his mental energy.

It is interesting to look at this case in the light of the interprofessional dementia model. Mr Smith is at the beginning of his dementia journey and, at this stage, primary care providers have important roles to play in identification of early cognitive impairment, in prevention and in early management, including support and education for the family. This is appropriately done in the social and environmental context of the patient's own home and community.

The NP reinforced this by visiting the patient and his wife in their own home, and conducting an initial assessment and early management of the patient in that setting. The focus is person and relationship centred, with education for both patient and carer, and management activities designed to fit in with the patient's lifestyle. This draws on the NP's professional and personal knowledge of the patient.

The case discussions demonstrated a number of subtle interplays between the personal and professional knowledge of the NP, the GP and the practice nurse. In the environment of a face-to-face discussion, roles and responsibilities could be decided, complexities – such as the cause-and-effect relationships between anxiety, depression and cognitive impairment in this man – discussed and a management plan agreed. This requires a good clinical understanding of dementia, collaborative skills and leadership skills. Good leadership recognises when to distribute tasks and responsibility and when to maintain control, and this was demonstrated by all participants: the GP, the practice nurse and the NP.

Conclusion

This chapter discussed leadership in the interprofessional team. An interesting focus of the leadership discussion was the focus on the leader's own personal strengths and weaknesses. As well as leading others, shaping systems, driving innovation and achieving outcomes, leaders need to be self-aware, and take opportunities for self-development. The case study illustrated this. The NP, while pioneering a new diagnostic and therapeutic role for nursing, also acted in a collaborative interprofessional way with GPs and others in case discussions. It was clear that the NP was willing to devolve responsibility as well as take it, and this is the essence of good leadership.

Self-directed learning activities

1 Who is taking the lead in this case study?
2 What leadership capabilities do you think are needed?
3 What collaboration is needed?
4 What part do other professionals and the patient take in the decision making?
5 Is the team working collaboratively?
6 What problems can you foresee occurring?

In addition to clear leadership, the team needs to be working in a collaborative way to ensure that it is effectively and efficiently providing care to the patient.

The following is an exercise you can carry out with your dementia care team to check whether effective collaboration is taking place.

Collaborative Working Survey

This survey is a diagnostic tool to take the pulse of the collaborative effort in a working team.

This will diagnose areas that are going well, as well as identifying areas where tensions exist. Tensions should be explored, through dialogue and reflective practice, to clarify the nature of difficulties and plan how to go forward.

The survey (Table 5.3) can be repeated over time to assess development and progress as the collaboration evolves.

Steps:

1 Distribute the survey to all members of the collaborative effort.
2 Ask each member individually to rate the extent they think the themes are present in the current collaborative working arrangements.
3 Collate the scores.
4 Present the collated scores to the group, highlighting areas that are strong, areas where there is a diverse range of views and areas where tensions seem to exist.

In following up responses from team members to the survey, these questions about the results might make for a productive conversation (adapted from Callahan et al., 2006):

1 What seem to be your strengths? (High percentages of colleagues agreeing that topics are both important and that they are currently happening.)
2 What might you conclude if there is a high percentage of 'disagree' ratings?
3 What does it mean when people regard an issue as important but feel it isn't currently happening? Follow-up questions include: *Why isn't it happening? What may need to be done about this?*
4 What does it mean when colleagues don't consider an issue very important?

What will you now do with the results?

TABLE 5.3 *Collaborative Working Survey*

STATEMENT TO ESTABLISH THE LEVEL TO WHICH COLLABORATION IS TAKING PLACE	DISAGREE	MODEST BEGINNING	CONSIDERABLE PROGRESS	FULLY AGREE
We have developed common aims	1	2	3	4
We have developed shared compatible aims	1	2	3	4
There is good communication between members	1	2	3	4
There is clarity about each member's role and who/what they represent	1	2	3	4
There are deepening bonds of commitment and determination between members to achieve the aims	1	2	3	4
Members are prepared to compromise in the interests of the common aims	1	2	3	4
We have developed effective working processes which helps get things done	1	2	3	4
There is accountability between members for following through on decisions which have been agreed	1	2	3	4
The leadership of the collaboration enacts principles of democracy and equality to empower everyone to take an active role	1	2	3	4
Members share resources	1	2	3	4
Members do not undermine each other or behave in ways which have a negative impact on others	1	2	3	4
Members trust each other to behave in ways which show respect	1	2	3	4
Power (personal and role) is used wisely to avoid over control by any one member	1	2	3	4
Due to working together we make faster, better decisions	1	2	3	4
Members share information and knowledge	1	2	3	4
Members are recognised and appreciated for their contribution	1	2	3	4
There is productive output as a result of our collaboration	1	2	3	4
The synergy achieved through collaboration makes things happen that wouldn't or couldn't otherwise	1	2	3	4
Individual total				

References

Alexopoulos, G.A., Abrams, R.C., Young, R.C. & Shamoian, C.A. (1988). Cornell scale for depression in dementia. *Biological Psychiatry Journal*. 23: 271–84.

Byrne, G.J. & Pachana, N.A. (2011). Development and validation of a short form of the Geriatric Anxiety Inventory – the GAI-SF. *International Psychogeriatrics*, 23(1): 125–31.

Callahan, C.M., Boustani, M.A., Unverzagt, F.W., Austrom, M.G., Damush, T.M., Perkins, A.J. … Hendrie, H.C. (2006). Effectiveness of collaborative care for older adults with Alzheimer disease in primary care: A randomized controlled trial. *Journal of the American Medical Association*, 295(18): 2148–57.

Health Workforce Australia (HWA). (2012). *Health Workforce 2015 Doctors, nurses and midwives* Volume 1. Retrieved 30 March 2015 from http://www.hwa.gov.au/sites/uploads/FinalReport_Volume1_FINAL-20120424.pdf

Health Workforce Australia (HWA). (2013). *Health LEADS Australia: The Australian Health Leadership Framework*. Adelaide: Health Workforce Australia.

Huppert, F.A., Brayne, C., Gill, C., Paykel, E.S. & Beardsall, L. (1995). CAMCOG – a concise neuropsychological test to assist dementia diagnosis: Socio-demographic determinants in an elderly population sample. *British Journal of Clinical Psychology*, 34: 529–41.

Logsdon, R.G., Gibbons, L.E., McCurry, S.M. & Teri, L. (2002). Assessing quality of life in older adults with cognitive impairment. *Psychosomatic Medicine*, 64(3): 510–19.

Oandasan, I., Baker, G.R., Barker, K., Bosco, C., D'Amour, D., Jones, L. … Way, D. (2006). *Teamwork in healthcare: Promoting effective teamwork in healthcare in Canada*. Ottawa: Canadian Health Services Research Foundation.

World Health Organization. (2010). *Framework for action on interprofessional education and collaborative practice*. Retrieved 30 March 2015 from http://www.who.int/hrh/resources/framework_ction/en/

6 Personal and professional knowledge

Dawn Forman and Jade Cartwright

Learning outcomes

1 Articulate the personal and professional attributes that may influence an individual's practice.

2 Discuss the course of dementia from health to illness to death.

3 Discuss the significance of the person's life lived before the onset of this disease.

4 Consider the impact of the journey of dementia on family and friends.

Key terms

- interprofessional

- personality

Introduction

In Chapter 1, we identified one key aspect of the Model of Interprofessional Practice and Education – Dementia (MIPPE-D) as being personal and professional knowledge. This capability looks at the practitioner as a whole, as well as the client, and recognises not only the professional knowledge that the individual brings to the situation but also their life skills, empathy and personal experiences.

What is personal knowledge?

In the previous chapters of this book, we have emphasised that every client is different and the importance for all health professionals to recognise their client's journey through life. We have also shown that health professionals need to develop background knowledge and skills to work in a professional and client-centred way.

However, we must also recognise that each professional will have had personal experiences outside their professional background. These will impact on how they see the world, how they react in situations and their values. They may, therefore, have a wide set of life skills that can be put into practice very effectively.

How does the individual professional know about the skills they possess and how to utilise them? In answering this, let's consider two aspects:

1 personality;
2 life skills.

> **Personality**
> Personality is made up of the characteristic patterns of thoughts, feelings and behaviours that make a person unique. It arises from within the individual and remains fairly consistent throughout life.

Personality

In the world of management theory, individuals are encouraged to understand their own **personality** first, in the belief that they who know themselves well, what their values are and the way in which they react in certain situations, will be better able to understand the way others will react.

De Haan and Burger (2004) outlined the structure of personality, which can be described as an onion, in Figure 6.1.

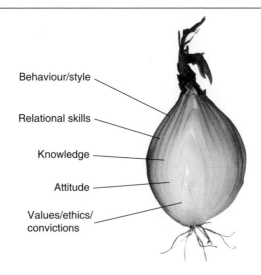

Behaviour/style

Relational skills

Knowledge

Attitude

Values/ethics/
convictions

FIGURE
6.1

A structure of personality (De Haan & Burger, 2004)
Reproduced with permission from De Haan & Burger.

They believe that values are developed over time as a result of experience and the influence of others. Behaviours can be more easily modified and developed, but all of these personality aspects can affect the interactions and engagements that take place with others.

Life skills

Life skills are the skills that we acquire through experience; some can be taught or encouraged but most are learnt through our experiences. Life skills are wide and varied but examples include:

- Employability skills;
- Transferable skills;
- Listening skills;
- Problem solving;
- Stress management;
- Social skills;
- Customer service skills;
- Parenting skills;

- Time management;
- Empathetic skills;
- Conflict resolution;
- Communication skills;
- Numeracy and literacy;
- Study skills;
- Financial skills;
- Anger management.

Applying personal skills to dementia care

When working in dementia care, a professional is often working closely with the individual and often over several years. This means that not only does the professional know the client very well but a trusting relationship has developed. Recognising when you need help not only on a professional basis but also on a personal basis can help you to help the client.

This simple checklist, modified from the one provided by the Family Caregiver Alliance (2015), can be used for any health care professional as well as the carer of a person with dementia:

1 *Set a positive mood for interaction.* Your attitude and body language communicate your feelings and thoughts more strongly than your words. Set a positive mood by speaking to the person with dementia in a pleasant and respectful manner. Use facial expressions, tone of voice and physical touch to help convey your message.

2   *Get the person's attention.* Limit distractions and noise – turn off the radio or TV, close the curtains or shut the door, or move to quieter surroundings. Before speaking, make sure you have their attention; address them by name, identify yourself by name, and use non-verbal cues and touch to help keep their focus. If seated, get down to their level and maintain eye contact.

3   *State your message clearly.* Use simple words and sentences. Speak slowly, distinctly and in a reassuring tone. Refrain from raising your voice higher or louder; instead, pitch your voice lower. If you are not understood the first time, use the same wording to repeat your message or question. If still not understood, wait a few minutes and rephrase the question. Use the names of people and places instead of pronouns or abbreviations.

4   *Ask simple, answerable questions.* Ask one question at a time; those with 'yes' or 'no' answers work best. Refrain from asking open-ended questions or giving too many choices. For example, ask, 'Would you like to wear your white shirt or your blue shirt?' Better still, show the choices – visual prompts and cues also help clarify your question and can guide a response.

5   *Listen with your ears, eyes and heart.* Be patient in waiting for a reply. If there is a struggle for an answer, it's okay to suggest words. Watch for non-verbal cues and body language, and respond appropriately. Always strive to listen for the meaning and feelings that underlie the words.

6   *Break down activities into a series of steps.* This makes many tasks much more manageable. You can encourage the person to do what they can, giving gentle reminders of steps that tend to be forgotten, and assisting with steps no longer accomplished independently. Using visual cues, such as showing with your hand where to place the dinner plate, can be very helpful.

7   *When the going gets tough, distract and redirect.* When the person becomes upset, try changing the subject or the environment. For example, ask for help or suggest going for a walk. It is important to connect with the person on a feeling level, before you redirect. You might say, 'I see you're feeling sad – I'm sorry you're upset. Let's go …' You can finish this sentence with '… get something to eat or drink or read' – whatever you feel is appropriate.

8   *Respond with affection and reassurance.* People with dementia often feel confused, anxious and unsure of themselves. Further, they often get reality confused and may recall things that never really occurred. Avoid trying to convince them that they are wrong. Stay focused on the feelings that they are demonstrating (which are real) and respond with verbal and physical expressions of comfort, support and reassurance. Sometimes holding hands, touching, hugging and praising will get the person to respond when all else fails.

9 *Remember the good old days.* Remembering the past is often a soothing and affirming activity. Many people with dementia may not remember what happened 45 minutes ago, but they can clearly recall their lives 45 years earlier. Therefore, avoid asking questions that rely on short-term memory, such as asking the person what they had for lunch. Instead, try asking general questions about the person's distant past – this information is more likely to be retained.

10 *Maintain your sense of humour.* Use humour whenever possible, though not at the person's expense. People with dementia tend to retain their social skills and are usually delighted to laugh along with you. (Modified with permission from Family Caregiver Alliance)

An **interprofessional** team can support not only the client but each of the professionals in the team. The following case study outlines a situation where various members of the interprofessional team need to consider not only their professional roles in helping the person with dementia but also how they pass information between each other.

> **Interprofessional**
> The terms 'interprofessional education/practice/ teamwork' etc. have been defined by various groups. These terms are often used interchangeably. Where we simply use the term 'interprofessional', we do so when two or more professions are working collaboratively together.

Knowing me, knowing you

Case study

Jade Cartwright, Curtin University, Australia

Marie is a speech pathologist with four years' clinical experience working in a range of hospital and community health care settings. Twelve months ago she joined a specialist dementia assessment and care unit that provides diagnostic assessment and management for people with dementia. The unit is made up of an interprofessional care team, including a neurologist and psychiatrist, clinical psychologists, neuropsychologists, social workers, occupational therapists and speech pathologists. The team regularly consults with community physiotherapists, dieticians, pharmacists and other health professionals on a needs basis.

Marie is currently working with a particularly complex client, Beth, a 78-year-old lady who lives at home alone in the community. Beth was widowed seven years earlier and her only daughter lives in London. She has a small group of friends whom she socialises with regularly. Beth presented to the unit with a three-year history of progressive speech difficulties, characterised by difficulty finding words and effortful, hesitant speech output. She was otherwise fit and healthy with no other medical complaints. She had described her symptoms to her GP on a number of occasions. However, she continued to perform well on the Mini Mental State Examination. She was referred to a specialist, but her symptoms were thought to be related to depression and anxiety associated with her husband's death. She was prescribed an antidepressant medication but her language symptoms persisted.

Beth remained certain that something more sinister was wrong and self-referred to the dementia assessment and care unit. She was seen by the team's neurologist and a neuropsychologist. Following extensive investigations and a series of cognitive assessments, a working diagnosis of primary progressive aphasia (PPA) was made. This diagnosis was met with some initial relief by Beth, providing as it did an explanation for her symptoms. However, she was upset to hear that the condition had no cure and was progressive in nature. Beth had not heard of aphasia or PPA before and was eager for more information about the condition.

PPA is a relatively rare dementia syndrome that targets the language networks of the brain (Mesulam, 1990; 2000). Symptoms are confined to the language domain for a period of at least two years, during which time individuals retain strong insight and awareness of their condition, and retain abilities in other areas of cognition such as memory, attention, visuospatial skills and executive functions (Mesulam, 2000). This was consistent with Beth's clinical presentation. She had acute insight into her speech difficulties, and remained independent in all activities of daily living that were not dependent on language. For example, she was able to clean, cook simple meals and complete personal care tasks independently, while continuing to manage all of her own financial affairs and medical appointments at home. She continued to drive and access the community without assistance. Beth's speech, however, was becoming progressively less fluent and effortful, with frequent word-finding hesitations. She described difficulties formulating language with sudden blockages, which she found incredibly frustrating. As a result, she was experiencing significant trouble speaking over the phone, running errands and making enquiries in the community, as well as participating in social conversation with her friends. Beth had made the decision not to talk to her daughter or friends about her diagnosis at that time as she did not want to worry or burden them.

After these initial appointments at the unit and receiving the diagnosis, Beth was referred for speech pathology assessment and ongoing management. Marie became Beth's case manager and was seeing Beth at home on a weekly basis to provide education and support. They quickly formed a strong rapport and Beth was thankful that Marie understood the nature of her speech difficulties and appreciated her genuine concern. Marie provided Beth with a range of word-finding strategies and communication aids, which Beth used willingly during speech sessions and conversations with Marie, with some positive effect. For example, Beth's written expression was more preserved than her verbal expression and she was often able to write words or short phrases that she was unable to say or recall verbally during conversation. Despite their effectiveness, Beth did not want to use these strategies in the community or with family and friends, and was attempting to mask her speech difficulties as much as possible.

About two months into their sessions, Marie was becoming increasingly worried about Beth's psychological status, suspecting that she was struggling to come to terms with her diagnosis. Beth had begun withdrawing from social interactions, was not eating and was losing weight. Beth also reported difficulty sleeping, and was lying awake at night worrying about her speech difficulties and the future. Beth acknowledged that she was embarrassed and ashamed of her speech difficulties, and felt that she was of little use to anyone if she was unable to talk. Beth was struggling to see that she had any residual strengths or positive qualities to draw upon.

Although Beth's primary symptoms and emotional reactions were related to her speech difficulties and PPA, Marie realised that she did not have the expertise to provide the counselling and support that Beth currently needed. Furthermore, Marie was starting to feel incredibly drained from the weight of Beth's concerns and was finding that she was lying awake at night herself trying to come up with practical solutions for her. As Beth's speech pathologist, Marie felt incredible pressure to support her client's communication and lessen the emotional distress that she was experiencing. Given the progressive nature of Beth's condition, Marie was also concerned for Beth's future and her psychological state in the long term.

This case scenario highlights some of the challenges that can be experienced by health professionals when working with clients with dementia, particularly with types of dementia that are less common or well-known. The scenario also supports current dementia policy advocating the need for timely diagnosis and early intervention, to help people come to terms with their diagnosis of dementia and to introduce proactive coping strategies to promote quality of life, while the search for a cure continues (Cubit & Meyer, 2011). Finally, while Beth presents with a focal dementia syndrome with primary speech concerns, her case highlights the critical need for a collaborative interprofessional approach, where health professionals work together to solve complex health care problems and optimise health outcomes (Keough & Huebner, 2000).

Getting to know yourself

While there are many personality tests that people can take to help get to know themselves better, the most powerful tool in a professional's armoury is refection.

During their education and training, professionals are asked to reflect on their experiences in practice and to learn from the mistakes that they make. In working with people with dementia, we strongly encourage professionals to reflect on their own reactions to situations. This reflection should include reflecting not only on what they did as a member of the health care team but also on their personality or personal values. For example, a situation may have made the professional annoyed or may have reminded them of a previous personal experience. A strong interprofessional team can help with this reflection in an informal way, as part of the team discussions, or in a more structured way, taking the form of action learning.

Action learning

Action learning was first developed by the physicist, Reg Revans. He found that talking through his problems to scientists of different disciplines enabled him to reflect more deeply about the situation he was facing and to derive for himself a different way forward. This encouragement to self-reflect on a situation is often used in coaching and is therefore often outlined as a coaching technique. Forman, Joyce and McMahon (2013) provided full guidance on how an action learning set can be developed, but in an interprofessional team it is helpful merely to encourage colleagues to take time to ask reflective, open questions, such as:

- How do you feel about the situation now?
- What do you remember thinking but not saying?
- What surprised you about the situation?
- Has this experience taught you anything about yourself, your assumptions, your values and your prejudices?
- What would you do differently next time?

By asking these questions, not only will the individual be reflecting on their personal reactions but the team will better understand each other and the person with dementia with whom they are working.

Conclusion

Knowing oneself and encouraging self-reflection on both personal and professional aspects of work is very helpful when working with a person with dementia, as the relationship is personal and develops over time.

Allowing personal reflections to be stimulated by open-ended questions, in the safe environment of an interprofessional group, will not only help professionals gain a deeper understanding of themselves and the others in the interprofessional team but will also help them to reflect on the person with dementia and how best to help them.

Self-directed learning activities

The following self-directed learning activities relate to the case study 'Knowing me, knowing you'. You may want to re-read this prior to looking at the questions below.

1   What does this scenario illustrate in terms of knowing the scope and limitations of one's own professional and personal roles, and responsibilities within a health care team?

2   What would you recommend as the next stage of management for Beth? How should Marie draw upon expertise within the interprofessional health care team?

3   Do you think it is important for Marie to reflect on how she is feeling in this scenario and her own approach to health care? Explain the reasons for your response.

4   What are some of the challenges health professionals may face when working with Beth, given her significant speech difficulties? How could these challenges be addressed in practice?

Case study

Julie was working with a group of professionals developing a shared care model of management for elderly war veterans suffering from cognitive impairment and post-traumatic stress disorder. The professionals consisted of Julie (a GP), Jane (a senior psychologist), Sarah (a postgraduate psychology student) and Louise (a social worker).

The model they developed involved identifying war veterans through general practice, and then involving them and their families in some structured therapy. After much discussion, during which each professional stated that they could alone deliver the whole package, the therapy was divided up into sessions. The war veteran sessions were to be delivered by the psychologist, sessions with the family to be delivered by the social worker, and some extra sessions on risky alcohol intake and medication reviews to be delivered by the GP. The psychology student was to make a manual of the psychology component of the work as part of her studies.

The team had some ongoing issues because of different personalities and agendas. The psychologist was very keen to have her student achieve an outcome, and was quite focused on evidence-based assessment and practice. She liked regular, scheduled meetings. The social worker was very client oriented and less concerned about structuring her part of the intervention too tightly. She often had trouble booking meetings ahead of time because of uncertainty about other commitments in her life. The GP tended to assume control of the situation at all times and all meetings were held in the GP's office.

About one year into the study, an argument developed in the team. Various psychological scales around cognitive function, anxiety and depression, and post-traumatic stress disorder had been finalised. Some team members were feeling quite satisfied with this result, when the social worker unexpectedly spoke up. 'All I ever hear about here is post-traumatic stress disorder, cognitive impairment and depression,' she said. 'I'm sick of it!' Other team members looked at her in surprise. 'Isn't that what we are on about?' they said.

'No, it is not!' said the social worker. 'What we are on about here is people! And these people have survived and lived their lives for many years, even with their post-traumatic stress disorder, depression and perhaps cognitive problems, and so have their families! Why don't we start looking at the positives – at the strengths of these people and their families?' She was very agitated and willing to get up and leave the project.

However, other members of the team wanted her to stay and explain. She fielded questions about a questionnaire to measure strengths, about how to measure outcomes from a strengths perspective and other issues that had never been considered by the more pathology focused team members. Eventually, the team came to understand that the strengths perspective was a valid one and would result in a different approach altogether. This approach was then incorporated to varying extents into different parts of the program.

Sadly, the money ran out before many people could be recruited. The team did receive a letter, though, from one of its few clients, saying that he was enormously grateful for the program, and only wished that he and his family had known about it when he was a younger man.

Reflective questions

1 Why was it important for the team to divide up the roles of the professionals into particular areas?
2 Might clear delineation of roles and responsibilities be necessary for good team functioning?
3 What problems might arise with this and how might they be resolved?
4 Why did some members of the team focus on pathology and others on strengths?
5 How might you assess the perspective of others in a team you are working on?
6 How much contribution might personality and personal agenda differences make to the team's 'brainstorming' episode?

Learning extension

In your interprofessional team, ask each person to think of any situation that they have experienced recently. In turn, allow five minutes for each person (the narrator) to outline the situation to the rest of the group. Using the questions outlined above and others that may occur to you, take it in turns to ask open-ended questions of the narrator. Those asking the questions should not attempt to interpret or say what they would do in the situation; they are merely helping the narrator to reflect, learn and find the next steps.

References

Cubit, K.A. & Meyer, C. (2011). Aging in Australia. *The Gerontologist*, 5(5): 583–9.

De Haan, E. & Burger, Y. (2004). *Coaching with colleagues: An action guide for one-to-one learning*. Basingstoke: Palgave Macmillan.

Family Caregiver Alliance. (2015). *Caregiver's guide to understanding dementia behaviours*. Retrieved 30 March 2015 from http://www.caregiver.org/caregivers-guide-understanding-dementia-behaviors

Forman, D., Joyce, M. & McMahon, G. (eds). (2013). *Creating a coaching culture for managers in your organisation*. London: Routledge.

Keough, J. & Huebner, R. (2000). Treating dementia: The complementing team approach of occupational therapy and psychology. *Journal of Psychology*, July 134(4): 375–91.

Mesulam, M.M. (1990). Large scale neurocognitive networks and distributed processing for attention language and memory. *Annals of Neurology*, 28: 597–613.

Mesulam, M.M. (2000). Behavioural neuroanatomy: Large-scale networks, association cortex, frontal syndromes, the limbic system and hemispheric specialization. In M.M. Mesulam (ed.) *Principles of behavioural and cognitive neurology* (pp. 1–120). New York: Oxford University Press.

7 Developing collaborative skills

Dawn Forman and Janet McCray

Learning outcomes

1   Review the collaborative skills required for interprofessional practice for people with dementia.

2   Consider how these skills are introduced into the working environment.

3   Discuss the factors that may affect staff resilience and the sustainability of good practice.

Key terms

- capabilities

- communication

- dementia

- interprofessional

- interprofessional collaboration (IPC)

- interprofessional teamwork

- resilience

- sustainability

- teamwork

Introduction

In Chapter 1, we looked at the competencies and capabilities that have been derived by various groups working in this area internationally. We noted that capability tools, to measure whether individuals in teams have these skills, continue to be developed and refined. In this chapter, we revisit these capabilities by asking how these could be introduced into an **interprofessional** team working with individuals who have **dementia** and how, with these skills, the team can become resilient to change and therefore can ensure an interprofessional culture that can be sustained by an organisation.

Interprofessional capabilities

There are a number of models and interprofessional capability tools that have been developed internationally. Interestingly, the same **capabilities** (with different emphases according to the country and the environment in which they have been developed) seem to be included in some way in these tools:

- client-centred;
- collaborative working;
- reflection;
- cultural awareness;
- organisational competence;
- leadership skills;
- communication;
- role clarification;
- professionalism;
- conflict resolution;
- ethics and values.

Even though tools already exist to measure collaborative skills, we need to create an environment in aged care settings that will help to cultivate them. We, therefore, need to ensure that an organisation is ready to have these skills introduced, staff are supported in their development and an environment is created that will support staff in both sustaining and enhancing them.

Creating the right environment

While the leaders and key stakeholders within the organisation will need to initiate the need for change, a novel approach has been developed by the Wicking Dementia Research and Education Centre in conjunction with the University of Tasmania. This model introduces students as change agents along with stakeholder facilitators.

The model presented in Figure 7.1, developed through the Wicking Teaching Aged Care Facility Program, sets out the key stages used. The

Interprofessional
The terms 'interprofessional education/practice/ teamwork' etc. have been defined by various groups. These terms are often used interchangeably. Where we simply use the term 'interprofessional', we do so when two or more professions are working collaboratively together.

Dementia
Dementia is now referred to as a neurocognitive disorder (NCD) (American Psychiatric Association, 2013), that is, the result of chronic or progressive damage to the brain.

Capabilities
Forman, Jones & Thistlethwaite (2014) define capability as 'has been used in preference to competence in one IPE framework, as it is considered by some educators to reflect more optimally the necessity that learners and professionals respond and adapt to health care and systems changes'.

Stage 1
Discovery
Preparation 5–6 months

- Organisational review of cultural dimensions including key stakeholder interviews/groups
- Design of change and communications approach
- Recruit mentor leader, identify mentor group and hold regular meetings to build capacity and develop resources
- Engagement of mentors in the unfamiliar process of researching their practice
- Benefits to success identified

Stage 2
Run-in
1st student placements

- Mentors facilitate placements with first student cohort
- Students & mentors participate in weekly meetings
- Data collection – pre/post test + qualitative
- Identification of key barriers to success
- Implementation of organisational processes and frameworks where possible in response to barriers

Stage 3
Review & strategy design

- Stakeholder workshops to design strategies in response to findings
- Program planning and scheduling
- Data analysis and reporting

Stage 4
Trial/prototype phase
2nd student placements

- Mentor-led implementation of revised interprofessional placements with a second cohort of students
- Ongoing coaching and support to organisational leaders about organisational cultural elements
- Capture of data from all stakeholders as trial progresses

Stage 5
Analysis & reporting

- Analysis of trial phase data
- Report of findings to the residential aged care facility and university stakeholders
- Organisational design elements to enable the establishment of a teaching nursing home implemented in line with discovery
- Benefits realisation measurement

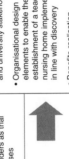

FIGURE 7.1 *A model for interprofessional teaching in aged care facilities (Robinson et al., 2014) Reproduced with permission from Robinson et al. from the Wicking Dementia Research and Education Centre, University of Tasmania.*

website (http://www.utas.edu.au/wicking) provides further information on this development and up-to-date resources on how to facilitate this change.

To ensure the sustained development of these skills, and thereby the continuity of effective teams, we need to ensure that the philosophy, policies and procedures are so embedded that these will exist, continue and develop even if there is a change of leadership. In research in this area, Micklan and Rodger (2005) undertook a study involving 202 health care professionals. Participants identified leadership as the most significant factor in maintaining **interprofessional teamwork** effectiveness. Sharing leadership functions was critical to the team's performance. Equally, as Cerra and Brandt (2011) noted, as the practice context is becoming more diverse, this may require new skill sets for effective team functioning.

> **Interprofessional teamwork** The levels of cooperation, coordination and collaboration characterising the relationships between professions in delivering patient-centred care.

Huxham and Vangen (2000) drew attention to the problem with all of the traditional leader/follower leadership models that incorporated a collaborative element. They noted the need for new leadership skills so that leaders can recognise the impact that these imposed processes and structures may have on themselves and their team, and learn to manage them, whilst devising tools to pursue, manage and shift an agenda forward. Leadership commitment is not only necessary from the top but from the team itself. For example, if one professional is absent in a multidisciplinary team, a key leadership role would be to ensure that resources are in place to provide the professional specific support required. In practice, this may require the leader to have political knowledge and strategies to fight for resources and lobby key players in economically tough times.

As Meads et al. (2009) stated, 'incorporating aspects of leadership, team working and resilience will help interprofessional development to be more sustainable in the future.'

Creating a consistent culture

Case study

Janet McCray, Chichester University, UK

Meadow Leigh is a 35-bedded residential home for adults with dementia. The home had a regular and reliable team of staff. However, a quality inspection highlighted a home in which residents, although physically well cared for, were observed as being disengaged. There was institutional practice with routines based around staff need rather than individual requirements. At the same time as the inspection, several other changes took place. The manager and two other full-time staff members left and a local day care service closed.

A new manager has arrived and is intent on providing person-centred care, and building up activity and engagement for the residents in and out of the home, with input from an interprofessional team including physiotherapists, occupational therapists, social workers, nurse specialists, rehabilitation care assistants, and volunteer and family members of the community. The manager has introduced new hours of working and is role-modelling new practice with the person at the centre. Focus is on the introduction of new activities and engagement of the clients. The manager has announced that two full-time staff will be replaced by part-time staff, and that commissioned, sessional input from specialists will be developed and evaluated, depending on resident need.

The original team of staff are unhappy and confused, and are responding negatively to the new options and incoming new interprofessional team members. Many of the original team know residents' family members and are expressing their views to them, creating tensions and distress, and suggesting residents will be unsettled.

Your role in the team

Person-centred practice consists of four key elements (Brooker, 2007):

1 working to a value base that values all irrespective of age or cognitive ability;
2 an individualised approach;
3 appreciating the world from the client's perspective;
4 providing a social environment that also fosters psychological needs.

Team-based care with the client at the centre holds five core principles (Mitchell et al., 2012):

1 shared goals;
2 clear roles;
3 mutual trust;
4 effective communication;
5 measurable processes and outcomes.

At Meadow Leigh, **communication** strategies and processes to embed this model may both impact on and be influenced by **interprofessional collaboration**. Hall (2005) observed that the stress and fatigue professionals feel in their collaborative settings may result in people retreating to their own individual professional silos. Team members will need an enhanced understanding of the work and roles that each member undertakes – and faces. Being able to share and model this understanding with family and other team

Communication
An exchange of information between individuals using speech, visual aids, body language, writing or behaviour.

Interprofessional collaboration (IPC) The process of developing and maintaining effective interprofessional working relationships with learners, practitioners, patients/clients/ families and communities to enable optimal health outcomes (Canadian Interprofessional Health Collaborative, 2010, p. 8).

members will help to build and promote positive responses to interprofessional team working and change.

Effective communication

Portner (2008, pp. 21–2) suggested a tendency in the field of older peoples' practice to be vague, to give unclear information and to use sophisticated, abstract, technical jargon hardly understandable to clients and other professionals. Openness and honesty in communication should be an aim from all professionals. At Meadow Leigh, the change to the delivery of care and personnel has implications for the nature of trust. Rowland (2013) described contrasts between personal and impersonal (or systems-oriented) trust. The previously established team at Meadow Leigh got on well and had personal trust. The new model of delivery will at least initially be dependent on impersonal or systems-oriented trust and could be vulnerable at stress points.

Some aspects of team work, created by changes outlined at Meadow Leigh, may result in a perceived division between the different professionals. As Collins and McCray (2012, p. 5) wrote 'interprofessional working has profound implications for practitioners, necessitating changes to working practices and the need to acquire new knowledge, skills, beliefs and identities.' (also in Cottrell & Bollom, 2007). Collins and McCray (2012) noted that, in a study exploring professional roles and identities, ambiguity and mistrust were expressed by practitioners from statutory and public services alike, regarding voluntary agencies' motivations and their adherence to professional codes around confidentiality and information sharing. At Meadow Leigh, there may be a lack of personal trust, of understanding of the challenges other professionals face, and of the confines in which they are working. Supporting and respecting all partners, and acknowledging the impact of changing boundaries on performance and deliverables, at the individual and team level, are critical. Delivering on stated practice goals, managing relationships through regular updates and feedback, and reflection and shared feedback on performance when intended outcomes are successful or less successful for the team will all need to be prioritised for communication to be effective.

Overcoming conflict and creating resilience

When services like Meadow Leigh are undergoing change, there is potential for considerable tension within interprofessional teams. One reason is because the balance of rewards and feedback available shifts, as priority is given to the accomplishment of team goals with the individual client. Initially motivation may be lower and stress levels higher. The impact of some forms of conflict, those that lead to discomfort and feelings of confusion, can, over time, create emotional problems, physical exhaustion, and dissatisfaction (Barber & Iwai, 1996). These factors clearly have a bearing on team **resilience** (West, Patera & Carsten, 2009) and how teams work. West, Patera & Carsten (2009) found that perceptions of team resilience were correlated positively with team cohesion, cooperation and coordination, and negatively with team conflict. Team resilience also correlated positively with team optimism and satisfaction (Delarue et al., 2008). In Meadow Leigh, strategies to address conflict, build positive practice models and create a culture of optimism are needed to ensure that changes made are sustainable.

> **Resilience**
> Individual resilience is the ability to bounce back from negative emotional experiences and flexible adaptation to the changing demands of stressful experiences (Tugade & Fredrickson, 2004).

Creating a sustainable, interprofessional culture

To achieve a positive sustainable, interprofessional culture, person-centred practice should drive processes. At Meadow Leigh, the team will need to determine and agree on models of practice to be used when dealing with conflict. Attention to the emotional resilience of the team may be required. This means determining how well the team copes in adverse conditions, and when to plan and deliver support to the team members. Team members will need to agree what a model of good **teamwork** practice and collaboration looks like. Equally, regular debriefing groups with the Meadow Leigh interprofessional team can be helpful when things work well and when they don't. Peer learning, using a coaching model, can help sustain good teamwork practice as part of collaboration in difficult situations. Zagenczyk et al. (2009, p. 240) observed that, in organisations where mentoring was offered, employees were more able to remain calm and positive for longer throughout difficult times.

> **Teamwork**
> Teamwork is the process of working collaboratively with a group of people in order to achieve a goal.

Leadership skills

In Meadow Leigh, the nature of the interprofessional team is changing and will shift dependent on the needs of the clients living in the home. Because of this not all traditional leadership models may be effective. Rowland (2013) suggested more in-depth exploration of leadership skills is required because of the fluidity of teams. In order to maintain effective teamwork and resilience among members at Meadow Leigh, different approaches may be required. One model that may fit is the Integrated Competing Values Framework (ICVF) (Vilkinas & Cartan, 2001; 2006). ICVF identifies six roles that are essential for leading any team (developer, innovator, broker, deliverer, monitor and integrator). Vilkinas and Cartan (2006) further identified that the leadership role needs to draw on the skills of each of the team members and integrate their contribution. Equally, Bolman and Deal's (2008) four frames of leadership that may be employed by team leaders (structural, human resource, political and symbolic) could also help. At Meadow Leigh, it is likely that the use of all four frames will be required to embed and sustain change.

Conclusion

In this chapter, we have reviewed the interprofessional capabilities required in an interprofessional team when working with a person with dementia. We have explored how these capabilities are introduced to an existing team, explored resilience in the teamwork setting and identified how interprofessional leadership education might be designed to promote **sustainability** within interprofessional and multidisciplinary working environments.

Sustainability
Sustainability is the endurance of systems and processes.

Self-directed learning activities

1 What would a person-centred team activity at Meadow Leigh involve?
2 How could you begin to establish trust among the team at Meadow Leigh?
3 What would positive teamwork behaviour include at Meadow Leigh?
4 How could you explore leadership models with the team at Meadow Leigh?

Learning extension

1 Revisit the competency/capability tools outlined in Chapter 1 to ensure that you are familiar with the skills needed for staff development.
2 Set out a plan for introducing these skills, developing staff and ensuring a sustainable environment for these interprofessional competencies.
3 Check out the Wicking Dementia Research and Education Centre website and think about whether this sort of model could be facilitated by your residential aged care facility and university working together.

References

Barber, C. & Iwai, M. (1996). Role conflict and role ambiguity as predictors of burnout among staff caring for elderly dementia patients. *Journal of Gerontological Social Work*, 26: 101–16.

Bolman, L.G. & Deal, T.E. (2008). *Reframing organisations: Artistry, choice and leadership* (4th edn). San Francisco: Jossey-Bass.

Brooker, D. (2007). *Person-centred dementia care: Making services better*. London: Jessica Kingsley.

Collins, F. & McCray, J. (2012). Partnership working in services for children: Use of the common assessment framework. *Journal of Interprofessional Care*, March 26(2): 134–40. doi: 10.3109/13561820.2011.630111.

Cottrell, D. & Bollom, P. (2007). Translating research into practice: The challenges of establishing a new multi-agency team for vulnerable children. *Journal of Children's Services*, 2(3): 52–63.

Cerra, F. & Brandt, C.F. (2011). Renewed focus in the United States links interprofessional education with redesigning health care. Guest editorial. *Journal of Interprofessional Care*, November, 25(6): 394–6. doi: 10.3109/13561820.2011.615576

Delarue, A., Van Hootegem, G., Procter, S. & Burridge, M. (2008). Teamworking and organisational performance: A review of survey-based research. *International Journal of Management Reviews*, June, 10: 127–48.

Hall, P. (2005). Interprofessional teamwork: Professional cultures as barriers. *Journal of Interprofessional Care*, (Supplement 1): 188–96.

Huxham, C. & Vangen, S. (2000). Leadership in the shaping and implementation of collaboration agendas: How things happen in a (not quite) joined-up world. *Academy of Management Journal*, 43: 1159–75.

Meads, G., Jones, I., Harrison, R., Forman, D. & Turner, W. (2009). How to sustain interprofessional learning and practice: Messages for higher education and health and social care. *Management Journal of Education and Work*, February, 22(1): 67–79.

Micklan, S.M. & Rodger, S.A. (2005). Effective health care teams: A model of six characteristics based on shared perceptions. *Journal of Interprofessional Care*, 19(4): 358–70.

Mitchell, P.M., Wynia, R., Golden, B., McNellis, S., Okun, C.E., Webb, V. . . . . Von Kohorn, I. (2012). Core principles and values of effective team-based health care. Discussion paper. Washington, DC: Institute of Medicine.

Portner, M. (2008). *Being old is different: Person-centred care for old people*. Ross-on Wye: PCCS Books.

Robinson, A., Lea, E., Tierney, L., See, C., Marlow, A., Morley, C.... Eccleston, C. (2014). *Teaching aged care facilities: Implementing interprofessional prevocational education and practice in residential aged care*. Hobart: Wicking Dementia Research and Education Centre, University of Tasmania. Retrieved 30 March 2015 from http://www.utas.edu.au/__data/assets/pdf_file/0010/525484/TACFP-Prevocational.pdf

Rowland, P. (2013). Core principles and values of effective team-based health care: A discussion paper. *Journal of Interprofessional Care*. doi: 10.3109/13561820. 2013.820906

Tugade, M.M. & Fredrickson, B.L. (2004). Resilient individuals use positive emotions to bounce back from negative emotional experiences. *Journal of Personality and Social Psychology*, 86: 320–33.

Vilkinas, T. & Cartan, G. (2001). The behaviour control room for managers: The integrator role. *Leadership and Organisational Development*, 22(4): 175–85.

Vilkinas, T. & Cartan, G. (2006). The integrated competing values framework: Its spatial configuration. *Journal of Management Development*, 25(6): 505–21.

West, B.J., Patera, J.L. & Carsten, M.K. (2009). Team level positivity: Investigating positive psychological capacities and team level outcomes. *Journal of Organisational Behaviour*, 30: 249–67.

Zagenczyk, T.J., Gibney, R., Kiewitz, C. & Restubog, S.D. (2009). Mentors, supervisors and role models: Do they reduce the effects of psychological contract breach? *Human Resource Management Journal*, 19(3): 237–59. doi: 10.1111/j.1748–8583.2009.00097

8 Person- and relationship-centred care in dementia

Kreshnik Hoti and Jeffery Hughes

Learning outcomes

1   Understand the principles of person-centred care of a person with dementia.

2   Understand who is the person in person-centred care.

3   Discuss approaches aimed at achieving person-centred care.

4   Understand the principles of relationship-centred care of a person with dementia.

5   Discuss the importance of the interprofessional team to collectively identify remaining abilities and the care pathway for the individual.

Key terms

● interprofessional practice (IPP)

● patient-focused care

● person-centred care

● relationship-centred care

Introduction

In this chapter, we discuss two key concepts involved in the care of patients with dementia: person-centred care and relationship-centred care. In addition to explaining the meaning and origins of person-centred care as a term, key emphasis is placed on principles and achievement of person-centred care. We also discuss the specifics of those with dementia that need consideration and the benefits of providing person-centred care in dementia patients. Relationship-centred care is explained in the context of interplay between collaboration, communication and relationships, and key interactions involved in dementia patients are also highlighted. We discuss relationships between various stakeholders involved in care of patients with dementia from the perspective of the agency theory. The chapter concludes with a consideration of interprofessional practice (IPP) in the provision of patient-centred care in dementia and the interprofessional team work is illustrated in a case study.

Person-centred care

Health care focused on the patient is increasingly becoming important for health policy makers around the world. The National Safety and Quality Framework, proposed by the Australian Commission on Safety and Quality in Health Care (ACSQHC), placed '**patient-focused care**' as the first of three areas needed to be addressed in order to achieve a safe and high quality health system in Australia (ACSQHC, 2009). Alzheimer's Australia, in their Position Paper 2 on quality of dementia care, indicated that high quality dementia care is achieved through person-centred care (Alzheimer's Australia, 2003).

> **Patient-focused care** Providing care that is respectful of and responsive to individual patient preferences, needs and values, and ensuring that patient values guide all clinical decisions.

The support for a health care system that focuses on the patient is strong in Australia with many providers embedding patient-focused principles into practice. A **person-centred care** focus is also popular internationally, especially in countries such as the US, UK and Canada.

Person-centred care is gaining more ground in dementia care and has evolved to become a synonym for good dementia care practice. The UK's National Institute for Health and Care Excellence (NICE) clinical guidelines highlight that person-centred care reflects good practice in dementia care, with many principles of person-centred care reflected in its guidelines (NICE, 2006). The term 'person-centred' care, although used in other health areas before, in dementia is relatively new. The term has its roots in the work of Carl Rogers and his 'client-centred' psychotherapy. According to Rogers, the aim is to create a setting so that the client can come up with their own resolution of their problems, rather than the therapist providing advice (Rogers, 1961; Lane, 2000). The term 'person-centred counselling' in fact replaced the 'client-centred' term, with the view of recognising that the person who seeks counselling is an expert on themselves, whereas the actual therapist is the facilitator who seeks the patient's self-actualisation (Brooker, 2004). However, it was not until

> **Person-centred care** Person-centred care is the 'treatment and care provided by health services which place the person at the centre of their own care and considers the needs of the older person's carers' (Victorian Government Department of Human Services, 2003).

the work of Kitwood that the 'person-centred' term found its way into dementia care (Kitwood, 1988; Kitwood, 1997). He supported the idea of shifting from the traditional approach of dementia care, which focused on the deficits of the person, to a model of care that values the personhood of the dementia patient. Kitwood emphasised that the term 'person-centred' care should be used with the view of highlighting communication and relationships during the process of dementia care (Kitwood, 1997). Dementia care mapping has been developed to assess the quality of care in dementia and is largely based on the person-centred care hence promoting patients' personhood and a holistic approach to their care.

Carers of dementia patients, who follow a person-centred care approach, bring out the best in the people living with dementia. This also applies to those care homes that often have their mission statement based around this approach and therefore aim to provide good dementia care. In this regard, it is worth emphasising that there are three key principles of good dementia care (Cheston, 1998; Kitwood, 1997):

- regular and structured activity;
- activity at interpersonal, recreational and therapeutic level;
- reinforcing patients' sense of worth and value.

What does person-centred care mean?

Brooker suggested that the term 'person-centred' care tends to mean different things to different people in various situations (Brooker, 2004). Therefore, articulating 'person-centred' care in a straightforward way is complex. To some, the term may imply individualised care; to others it is a value base. This is also obvious from various approaches that regard 'person-centred' care as a set of techniques of working with a patient with dementia in comparison to other approaches in which 'person-centred' care is based on communication with the patient (Brooker, 2004). It should also be recognised that, in practice, the person-centred care term is used interchangeably with terms such as 'personalised care', 'patient-centredness' and 'relationship-centred care'. Overall, the term describes the relevance of relationships and collaboration between health care workers and patients and recognises their needs and reciprocity in relationships (ACSQHC, 2010). As a concept, person-centred care puts the patient first. This essentially means putting patients' needs, feelings, preferences, experiences and well-being ahead of the disease, in this case dementia. Therefore, person-centred care is entirely and always focused on the individual person.

There are a number of definitions of person-centred care but none is currently globally accepted. One of the definitions provided by the Victorian Government Department of Human Services (2003) defines person-centred care as 'treatment and care provided by health services which place the person at the centre of their own care and considers the needs of the older person's carers'. This definition also considers the carers (i.e. service providers) and emphasises the importance of the collaborative and respectful partnership that should be in place between carers and patients (i.e. service providers and users). According to the Institute for Patient- and Family-Centred Care (n.d.), person-centred care:

> is an innovative approach to the planning, delivery, and evaluation of health care that is grounded in mutually beneficial partnerships among health care providers, patients, and families. Patient- and family-centred care applies to patients of all ages, and it may be practised in any health care setting.

The World Health Organization (WHO) used the term 'responsiveness' over 'person-centred care' with the view of best describing how health care systems meet expectations in a number of domains, namely respect for people and their preferences, communication between healthcare workers and patients, as well as waiting times (WHO, 2000). WHO also supports carer and patient involvement in partnership initiatives with the aim of improving safety and quality of care (WHO, 2010).

In recognising, therefore, that 'person-centred' care is a composite term, Brooker (2007) proposed that in dementia care it should encapsulate four major components referred to as VIPS:

- valuing people with dementia and those who care for them (V);
- treating people as individuals (I);
- looking at the world from the perspective of the person with dementia (P);
- providing a positive social environment in which the person living with dementia can experience relative well-being (S).

Achieving person-centred care

According to the UK's Royal College of Nursing (n.d.), there are some key considerations that assist individual carers in the achievement of person-centred care. These considerations are based on concepts that need to ensure:

- respect and holism;
- power and empowerment;

- choice and autonomy;
- empathy and compassion.

In general, there are a number of approaches reported internationally that assist in achieving person-centred care. These include a variety of strategies generally aimed at improving patients' knowledge (e.g. through training of health professionals about medicines and longer consultation times for patients); improving patients' experience (e.g. getting patient feedback through surveys that support quality improvements, person-centred communication and longer consultation times); improving service use and decreasing cost (e.g. public reporting of performance, adequate dissemination of information in formats easily understood by patients) and improving health behaviour and health status (e.g. through development of communication skills for clinicians) (ACSQHC, 2010; Coulter & Ellins, 2006).

Engagement of carers and patients is a cornerstone in achieving person-centred care. The relevance of carers and/or family should be highly valued given their knowledge of the patient (e.g. history and routines) and their ability to reassure the patient in various situations of uncertainty, anxiety or even vulnerability. Carer involvement in patients' care can be supported by designing strategies aimed at readjusting patient visiting times according to their needs, creating family response teams that alert health care staff on changes in patients' status and creating partnerships with carers and/or families aimed at addressing patients' needs (ACSQHC, 2010). Such strategies can contribute to the overall care of the patient and improve their overall experience as suggested by Frampton et al., (2008) who reported a 65% decrease in anxiety and improved overall patient experience as a result of patient-directed visiting hours.

Access to information and education by carers and patients is also a person-centred strategy that promotes empowerment. In this regard, patient personalised information, provision of printed and electronic information, as well as educational programs, improve knowledge and understanding of their condition and hence benefit patients' care (Frampton et al., 2008; ACSQHC, 2010).

Approaches aimed at improving the design of the physical care environment for patients by creating a user-centred design have also been reported to be successful in improving patients' experience of care. Service re-design has also been implemented in this context in the UK. This approach focuses on technical issues of the patient's journey and it maps steps in order to identify potential problems in the patient's care and hence generates solutions (Ben-Tovim et al., 2008).

Appointing carers and patients to advisory committees at governance level, in order to have a say in decision-making processes, is also important in ensuring person-centred care. This strategy can assist by having carers and patients providing information to policy makers on their needs and concerns, being involved in planning of patient care and innovative programs, having their say on changes affecting patients and carers, and helping to strengthen communication between various stakeholders in the patient care chain (i.e. family, carers, health care staff, administrative staff and patients). Appointment of carers and patients at governance level also encourages them to speak up and get involved in the care process (ACSQHC, 2010; Frampton et al., 2008).

Important considerations in achieving person-centred care also include ensuring that care providers offer an environment that supports person-centred care. In addition to creating an atmosphere that supports patient-centredness, providers should consider staff satisfaction and accountability strategies, as well as valuing training and ensuring that employees' behaviour in fact reflects the organisation's values (Shaller, 2007; Frampton et al., 2008).

Person-centred care in dementia

Who is the person?

Patients with dementia have unique characteristics owing to their disease. Dementia imposes various levels of functional decline (both physical and cognitive). Its progressive nature in relation to cognition, behaviour, as well as function tends to make patients with dementia more dependent on other people, especially in the performance of activities of daily living (Chenoweth et al., 2009). This translates into unmet complex needs of patients with dementia leading to behaviours that are need-driven (Chenoweth et al., 2009; Kitwood, 1997). Behavioural and psychological symptoms of dementia (BPSD), also referred to as neuropsychiatric symptoms, are a diverse group of non-cognitive symptoms and behaviours that occur in patients with dementia (Cerejeira, Lagarto & Mukaetova-Ladinska, 2012). These symptoms correlate with the degree of functional and cognitive impairment. Delivery of care in dementia patients is therefore often complicated by the presence of BPSD, which includes agitation, aberrant motor behaviour, anxiety, elation, irritability, depression, apathy, disinhibition, delusions, hallucinations, and sleep or appetite changes (Cerejeira, Lagarto & Mukaetova-Ladinska, 2012).

These issues place carers in difficult and stressful positions, and also lead to distress and institutionalisation of patients with dementia. Therefore, there are specific issues that should be considered when providing, or aiming to provide, person-centred care. The degree of care provision is dependent upon the individual with dementia. This process is driven by the carers' ability to observe the person's expression of well-being and, based on that, ability to evaluate the degree of person-centred care to be offered. This detailed observation and evaluation of a person's well-being by carers assists during the process of planning, implementation and assessment of person-centred care (Chenoweth et al., 2009).

Principles of person-centred care in dementia

In achieving person-centred care, there are several considerations to follow in dementia care (Alzheimer's Society, (n.d.); Alzheimer's Australia, 2003; NICE, 2006). These include:

- viewing the person as an individual – this means shifting the focus from their disease as well as lost abilities as a result of their disease;
- viewing the person as a whole – this means considering the individual person's preferences, interests, needs, qualities and abilities instead of focusing solely on managing their symptoms;
- making the person an equal partner in health care – this involves empowering the patient in the decision-making processes around their health;
- getting to know the person – this means knowing about the person's life, history, family and values;
- treating the person with dementia with dignity and respect – this involves recognising and encouraging the person's unique strengths during their management and treating them with courtesy at all times;
- taking into account the person's cultural and religious beliefs.

In addition to the above individual considerations that assist dementia carers in achieving person-centred care, the Health Foundation (n.d.) outlines that person-centred care can only be achieved when:

- Staff possess adequate knowledge and skills to provide person-centred care.
- There are systems and processes designed to facilitate staff to act in a person-centred manner, and respond to service users' needs and preferences.
- People who use and those who provide the service, co-design and co-produce it, enable support for person-centred care.

In 2010, the Victorian Department of Health issued keys to delivering person-centred care for persons with dementia in their publication regarding good practice for dementia care. These are summarised in Table 8.1.

TABLE 8.1 *Keys to person-centred care (Modified from the Victorian Government Department of Human Services, 2010)*

PERSON WITH DEMENTIA	CARERS
Care should understand the person's behaviour in relation to their unmet needs	Carer–person relationship is the key
Care should not be physical focused only and it should involve the whole person, including their social, cultural and individual identity	Carer has good information about the person during their care and shares this information with the management in order to develop appropriate strategies
Care should acknowledge person's unique interests and life stories	Carers are in touch with their own concerns and feelings
Care should acknowledge person's abilities, interests, preferences, values and spirituality	All staff are able to become experts in dementia care

Why person-centred care?

A person-centred care approach reduces behavioural and psychological symptoms of dementia patients, and it also facilitates maintenance of patients' personhood (Edvardsson, Winblad & Sandman, 2008). Person-centred care not only enables the person to become a partner of the interprofessional health care team, but also a key driver enabling the achievement of the best health outcomes for the person. In general, person-centred care provides benefits in terms of care experience as well as operational benefits. Engagement of various stakeholders (e.g. health care providers, patients, families) in care based on partnerships results in better quality and safety of health services provided, decreased cost and increased satisfaction of patients and other stakeholders involved (ACSQHC, 2010). Decreased length of hospital stay, decreased staff vacancy rates and an increased rate of hospital discharges have also been reported as a result of the person-centred approach (Stone, 2008).

Literature has also reported that person-centred care results in decreased infection rates and medication errors (DiGioia, n.d.), and improved clinical care (Jha et al., 2008) and functional status (Flach et al., 2004). Improved chronic disease management has also been reported (Stewart et al., 2000; Bauman, Fardy & Harris, 2003).

Specific clinical benefits of a person-centred care approach in patients with dementia have also been reported. These benefits can be non-pharmacological and pharmacological in nature (e.g. reduced agitation and anxiety as well as reduced use of antipsychotic medications). The Caring for Aged Dementia Care Resident Study (CADRES), which was a cluster randomised clinical trial of 324 people with dementia, reported that as an intervention, person-centred care significantly improved agitation compared to usual care (Chenoweth et al., 2009). A reduction in agitation of nursing home residents was also reported by Cohen-Mansfield, Libin and Marx (2007) through the introduction of a personalised care technique based on individual residents' needs (Cohen-Mansfield, Libin and Marx, 2007). In addition to agitation, anxiety can also be reduced through staff training on person-centred care in relation to specific individualised bathing practices for patients with dementia.

Similarly, a reduction in use of antipsychotic medications for the management of behavioural and psychological symptoms of residents with dementia has also been reported in a cluster randomised study by Fossey et al. (2006). The use of antipsychotic medication in patients with dementia is still a debatable and complex issue as their benefits are modest at best for these patients and their use is justified only in limited situations. Approximately 80% of people with dementia receive antipsychotic medication for behavioural and psychological symptoms (Hosia-Randell & Pitkälä, 2005). Antipsychotics use in people with dementia has a number of adverse effects leading to deterioration of health and, furthermore, is associated with an increased mortality in this patient group. A recent Alzheimer's Australia report titled *The Use of Restraints and Psychotropic Medications in People with Dementia* has highlighted the negative consequences of using antipsychotics in patients with dementia, including the fact that these drugs are not always appropriately prescribed with evidence suggesting their misuse in patients with dementia (Peisah & Skladzien, 2014). Therefore, as also highlighted in Figure 8.1, a person-centred care approach may reduce dementia patients' mortality through reduction of behavioural and psychological symptoms, such as agitation and anxiety, and reduction of antipsychotic medication use.

Relationship-centred care

The importance of relationships and interactions to persons with dementia is clearly articulated in NICE guidelines (2006) reflecting good practice care in dementia. It is an imperative in dementia care to recognise the needs of carers, and to also consider ways of supporting and enhancing their input to the

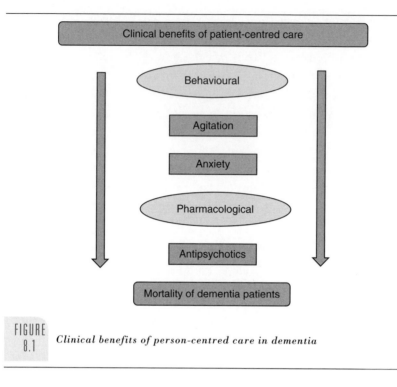

FIGURE
8.1 *Clinical benefits of person-centred care in dementia*

person with dementia (NICE, 2006). Beach and colleagues argue that there are a number of functions that take place within the context of relationships and these include information exchange, diagnosing, prescribing (i.e. choosing treatment), resource allocation and assessment of care outcomes (NICE, 2006). In the general context, these authors propose that relationship-centred care is built upon four major principles:

1 Relationships in health care ought to include dimensions of personhood as well as roles. This principle acknowledges the fact that health care providers and patients have their own experiences, emotions and values, which should be recognised.

2 Affect and emotion are important components of relationships in health care. This principle acknowledges the need for health care providers being encouraged to empathise with the patient. Affect and emotion are, in fact, central to developing, maintaining and terminating relationships.

3 All health care relationships occur in the context of reciprocal influence. This principle acknowledges the interactional exchange between health care providers and patients. This principle points out that the relationship

should not be one between unequals, where health care providers are the 'experts', but rather reciprocal and based on attainment of virtue.

4 **Relationship-centred care** has a moral foundation.

The value of relationships in the context of person-centred care in dementia has been emphasised and initially articulated by Kitwood (1997), who used the term by emphasising communication and relationships during the process of dementia care. It can be argued that person-centred care is a by-product of nurtured and reciprocal relationships, close collaborations and effective communications between health care workers and carers involved in the care process, including the person (Figure 8.2).

> **Relationship-centred care**
> Relationship-centred care is care in which all participants appreciate the importance of their relationships with one another (Beach, C., Inui, T. & the Relationship-Centred Care Research Network, 2006).

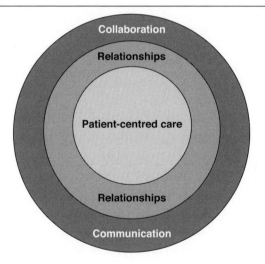

FIGURE 8.2 *Interplay of collaboration, communication and relationships in person-centred care*

Patients with dementia are key stakeholders in health care delivery and their effective collaboration with health care providers is established on their strong relationship and ultimately mutual trust. Of great importance is also the relationship between various health care providers with diverse expertise, as well as the relationship between these health care providers and dementia carers, including family. These relationships are nurtured by effective collaboration for the patient with dementia. In fact, the relationship is also dependent on collaboration outcomes.

Collaboration and, therefore, relationships between health care providers are of high importance in **IPP**. Previous studies have reported that relationships between health care teams have direct benefits on patient outcomes (mortality ratios) (Knaus et al., 1986; Zillich et al., 2004). Theoretical frameworks have been developed to evaluate the doctor–pharmacist relationship. Models, such as the Collaborative Working Relationship and the Pharmacist–Physician Collaborative Index, were developed to evaluate the extent of collaborative relationships of health professionals (McDonough & Doucette, 2001; Snyder et al., 2010). While these models assist in assessing the relationship, the agency theory can assist in understanding the relationship between the patient with dementia (i.e. principal), as well as health care providers and carers (agents), who in fact perform actions (as agents) on behalf of the patient (the principal). The agency theory was used in the context of drug selection by Mott, Schommer, Doucette and Kreling (1998) and then in the area of prescribing by Hoti, Hughes and Sunderland (2011) and Hoti, Forman and Hughes, 2014. Its principles can be applied in dementia care given that the theory predicts that information asymmetry is reduced when agents have more information about their principal. This is relevant in person-centred care since one of the reported strategies to person-centred care relies on the information that carers and health care providers have about the patient with dementia that assists in care planning (e.g. history, routine) (ACSQHC, 2010).

Interprofessional practice (IPP)
Occurs when all members of the health service delivery team participate in the team's activities and rely on one another to accomplish common goals and improve health care delivery, thus improving the patient's quality experience (Australasian Interprofessional Practice and Education Network, 2011).

While recognising that relationships between health care providers are important, in relationship-centred care the relationship between the patient and health care providers is central (Beach, Inui & the Relationship-Centered Care Research Network, 2006). In dementia care, relationship is closely affiliated with interaction between the patient and carers, and clearly in person-centred care there is a special focus on the interaction, and hence relationship, between the person and people involved in their care. In this regard, Kitwood (1997) identified 10 types of interactions specifically related to dementia care:

1 *Recognition* involves acknowledging the person with dementia such as greeting by name.
2 *Negotiation* involves acknowledging and consulting dementia patients' preferences.
3 *Collaboration* involves carers and patients with dementia working together.
4 *Play* involves allowing patients with dementia to express themselves and be spontaneous.

5 *Simulation* is an interaction in which senses are the key focus. In this context it means sensuous or sensual interaction, which includes aromatherapy and massage.

6 *Celebration* is an interaction that involves experiencing the joy of carers and patients with dementia.

7 *Relaxation* is an interaction that involves provision of an environment enabling relaxation.

8 *Validation* involves recognising feelings and emotions of patients with dementia, and responding at an appropriate level.

9 *Holding* involves providing a safe psychological space enabling expression of dementia patients' feelings such as grief, anger or fear.

10 *Facilitation* involves interaction that enables the patient with dementia to do things that they are not otherwise able to do as a result of their functional or cognitive decline.

Interprofessional consideration of person-centred care in dementia

As highlighted above, care of patients with dementia is complex, with its own characteristics due to the progressive nature of the disease and the array of symptoms, functional and cognitive disabilities displayed. Care needs to address a range of daily living activities, including mobility, toileting, oral health, grooming and safety. There is also a range of discomforts, including pain, incontinence, malnutrition and drug misadventures, such as adverse effects and drug interactions (Edvardsson, Winblad & Sandman, 2008; Nair, 2006). Patients with dementia also have a spectrum of psychological basic human needs, including feeling of safety, sense of belonging and acceptance, socialisation, need to be respected and sense of contribution. (Edvardsson, Winblad & Sandman, 2008) The above specifics of dementia care highlight the need for involvement of multiple health care teams with diverse expertise in the cycle of dementia care. In this regard, an IPP approach is crucial given that it improves effectiveness and safety of care (Chapter 2 of Greiner & Knebel, 2003). IPP is a partnership that involves care delivery by a range of diverse health care workers working collaboratively, with a focus on the patient, while sharing the decisions and overall care of the patient (Canadian Interprofessional Health Collaborative, 2010). Uniprofessional health care delivery is becoming increasingly less viable, given the rise in prevalence of chronic conditions (Dunston et al., 2009). Dementia too is projected to increase in prevalence, with numbers in Australia estimated to increase by one third in less than 10 years to 400000 cases and with *World Alzheimer's Report 2010* estimating a rise from the current 36 million global cases to 115 million by 2050 (Alzheimer's Australia, 2003; Wimo & Prince, 2010). Australian health providers are increasingly recognising and employing IPP as a way of delivering person-centred care (Steketee et al., 2014). Tertiary education providers are also placing an emphasis on interprofessional education (IPE) for health students. Successful integration of students in IPE teams and positive student experiences with an attitudinal shift towards IPE and IPP have also been reported (Hoti, Forman & Hughes, 2014).

Person-centred care interventions, resulting in both pharmacological and non-pharmacological benefits, are important from the IPE and practice point of view as they allow integration of an increased number of health practitioners with varying expertise within interprofessional teams, including nurses, psychologists, doctors, occupational therapists, speech pathologists, physiotherapists and pharmacists. A more detailed discussion of the integration of these health practitioners in interprofessional teams is given in the following case study.

Case study

Thelma is a 79-year-old lady diagnosed with Alzheimer's disease two years ago. Over the last couple of months, her condition has deteriorated with Thelma not being able to perform most of her basic daily activities. She was admitted to Harmony Keys Nursing Home two weeks ago, after her daughter Brenda, who is also her full-time carer, found it increasingly difficult and stressful to manage her mum on her own, especially her toileting and bathing. Prior to being diagnosed, Thelma also suffered from osteoarthritis, hypertension and incontinence.

Thelma's current medications are displayed in the table below.

Ramipril 5mg tablets	1 in the morning
Aspirin 100mg tablets	1 in the morning (refuses to take)
Paracetamol 500mg tablets	1 twice daily
Docusate 50mg, with Senna 8mg tablets	2 in the evening
Donepezil 5mg tablets	1 in the morning

At 2 am, Brenda was called by carers of the nursing home as Thelma became very agitated, and was suffering delusions and hallucinations. They called her to see if she remembered her mother having similar behaviours before. Today, Thelma is still agitated, although her delusional behaviour and hallucinations seem to have settled.

The Harmony Keys Nursing Home has recently adopted an IPP policy and, as a result of this practice, Thelma is today being assessed by an interprofessional team consisting of a doctor, nurse, pharmacist, physiotherapist and speech pathologist.

There are two key questions about Thelma's care pathway that currently arise from the team:

1 What profession-specific recommendations can be made for Thelma's current situation?
2 What would an interprofessional care plan for managing Thelma's current situation consist of?

The interprofessional team management

Case study:

Profession-specific recommendations would vary, given the diverse expertise of the doctor, nurse, pharmacist, physiotherapist and speech pathologist. From an IPP point of view, it is the prioritisation of recommendations (i.e. interventions) that becomes of crucial importance for Thelma's care. Involving Brenda is also important as it is one of the steps needed to deliver person-centred care for Thelma. This is the first time that Thelma has experienced these symptoms; therefore, the information that Brenda, her daughter and long-time carer, provides is highly relevant. After consulting Brenda, the team finds out that Thelma has never displayed this sort of behaviour at home and that she does not like taking multiple tablets. Each professional undertakes their own assessments then presents their findings to produce an interprofessional care plan, as shown in Figure 8.3.

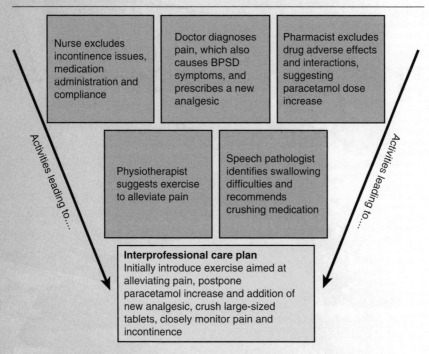

Nurse excludes incontinence issues, medication administration and compliance

Doctor diagnoses pain, which also causes BPSD symptoms, and prescribes a new analgesic

Pharmacist excludes drug adverse effects and interactions, suggesting paracetamol dose increase

Physiotherapist suggests exercise to alleviate pain

Speech pathologist identifies swallowing difficulties and recommends crushing medication

Activities leading to....

Activities leading to....

Interprofessional care plan
Initially introduce exercise aimed at alleviating pain, postpone paracetamol increase and addition of new analgesic, crush large-sized tablets, closely monitor pain and incontinence

FIGURE 8.3 *Development of an interprofessional approach from profession-specific findings for Thelma's current complaint*

From Figure 8.3, we can see that Thelma's behavioural and psychological symptoms in dementia symptoms are being caused by undiagnosed or undertreated pain. Some of the profession-specific recommendations, such as increasing paracetamol dose or adding a new analgesic, although relevant, are therefore not included in the current actions in the interprofessional care plan to manage Thelma's pain.

By working collaboratively, the health care team is informed and their final recommendations influenced by each other when designing an interprofessional plan (e.g. increasing the number of paracetamol tablets to reach the optimum dose, or changing it to a higher slow release formulation, becomes less attractive as a first choice given that the speech therapist has recommended crushing medications).

In a person-centred approach, which includes the patient's carer/family and also considers the person's needs and preferences, information provided may also influence the interprofessional decision-making process (i.e. Thelma does not like taking multiple medications, which can also influence the decision as to whether to increase the paracetamol dose or add a new analgesic, in addition to other clinical reasons such as potential adverse effects).

Conclusion

This chapter has emphasised the relevance of providing person-centred care and relationship-centred care in patients with dementia. The achievement of patient care is described through revisiting key principles and interactions involved in achieving person-centred care. An interprofessional model designed and trialled in practice has been provided to illustrate the integration of various members of the health care team while ensuring that the patient remains the focus of interprofessional care.

Self-directed learning activities

1 How would you achieve person-centred care at Harmony Keys Nursing Home?
2 What key activities would you consider, both profession-specific and inter-professional, while ensuring patient-centred care is maintained at Harmony Keys Nursing Home?
3 How could you strengthen collaboration within a nursing home with a view to providing patient- and relationship-centred care?

Learning extension

1 Review the principles recommended in the provision of person-centred care.

2 Check out the recommended websites to further explore the relevance of person-centred care in patients with dementia.

3 Consider the interprofessional model described in this chapter, and the advantages of and barriers to applying a similar model in your residential aged care facility (RACF).

4 Review the characteristics of patients with dementia in your RACF and consider how these characteristics affect the provision of patient-centred care.

References

Alzheimer's Australia. (2003). *Quality of dementia care.* Retrieved 14 August 2014 from http://www.fightdementia.org.au/

Alzheimer's Society. (n.d.). Definition of person-centred care. Retrieved 15 August 2014 from http://www.alzheimers.org.uk/

Australian Commission on Safety and Quality in Health Care (ACSQHC). (2009) *National safety and quality framework – a national framework for improving the safety and quality of health care.* Retrieved 12 August 2014 from http://www. safetyandquality.gov.au/

Australian Commission on Safety and Quality in Health Care (ACSQHC). (2010). *Person-centred care: improving the quality and safety by focusing care on patients and consumers.* Retrieved 11 August 2014 from http://www.safetyandquality.gov.au/

Bauman, A., Fardy, H. & Harris, P. (2003). Getting it right: Why bother with person-centred care? *Medical Journal of Australia,* 179: 253–6.

Beach, C., Inui, T. & the Relationship-Centred Care Research Network. (2006). Relationship-centred care: A constructive reframing. *Journal of General Internal Medicine,* 21(Supplement 1): S3–S8.

Ben-Tovim, D., Dougherty, M., O'Connell, T. & McGrath, K.M. (2008). Patient journeys: The process of clinical re-design. *Medical Journal of Australia,* 188: S14–S17.

Brooker, D. (2004). What is person-centred care in dementia? *Clinical Gerontology,* 13: 215–22.

Brooker, D. (2007). *Person-centred dementia care: Making services better.* London: Jessica Kingsley Publishers.

Canadian Interprofessional Health Collaborative. (2010). *A national interprofessional competency framework.* Retrieved 25 July 2014 from http://www.cihc.ca

Cerejeira, J., Lagarto, L. & Mukaetova-Ladinska, E.B. (2012). Behavioural and psychological symptoms of dementia. *Frontiers in Neurology*, 3: 73.

Chenoweth, L., King, M.T., Jeon, Y.H., Brodaty, H., Stein-Parbury, J., Norman, R. … Luscombe, G. (2009). Caring for Aged Dementia Care Resident Study (CADRES) of person-centred care, dementia-care mapping, and usual care in dementia: A cluster-randomised trial. *Lancet Neurology*, 8(4): 317–25.

Cheston, R. (1998). Psychotherapeutic work with people with dementia: A review of the literature. *The British Journal of Medical Psychology*, 71: 211–31.

Cohen-Mansfield, J., Libin, A. & Marx, M. (2007). Non-pharmacological treatment of agitation: A controlled trial of systematic individualised intervention. *Journals of Gerontology Series A: Biological Sciences and Medical Sciences*, 62: 908–16.

Coulter, A. & Ellins, J. (2006). *Patient-focused interventions: A review of the evidence.* Oxford: Picker Institute Europe.

DiGioia, A.M. (n.d.). *The AHRQ Innovation Exchange: Patient- and family-centred care initiative is associated with high patient satisfaction and positive outcomes for total joint replacement patients.* Retrieved 1 August 2014 from https://innovations.ahrq.gov/

Dunston, R., Lee, A., Matthews, L.R., Nisbet, G., Pockett, R., Thistlethwaite, J. & White, J. (2009). *Interprofessional health education in Australia: The way forward.* Sydney: University of Sydney and the University of Technology Sydney, Australian Learning and Teaching Council.

Edvardsson, D., Winblad, B. & Sandman, P.O. (2008). Person-centred care of people with severe Alzheimer's disease: Current status and ways forward. *Lancet Neurology*, 7(4): 362–7.

Flach, S.D., McCoy, K.D., Vaughn, T.E., Ward, M.M., Bootsmiller, B.J. & Doebbeling, B.N. (2004). Does patient-centred care improve provision of preventive services? *Journal of General Internal Medicine*, 19: 1019–26.

Fossey, J., Ballard, C., Juszczak, E., James, I., Alder, N., Jacoby, R. & Howard, R. (2006). Effect of enhanced psychosocial care on antipsychotic use in nursing home residents with severe dementia: Cluster randomised trial. *British Medical Journal*, 332: 756–61.

Frampton, S., Guastello, S., Brady, C., Hale, M., Horowitz, S., Bennett Smith, S. & Stone, S. (2008). *The patient-centred care improvement guide.* Derby, CT: Planetree in collaboration with Picker Institute.

Greiner, A.C. & Knebel, E. (2003). *Health professions education: A bridge to quality.* Washington, DC: National Academies Press.

Health Foundation. (n.d.). Definition of person-centred care. Retrieved 15 August 2014 from http://www.health.org.uk

Hosia-Randall, H. & Pitkälä, K. (2005). Use of psychotropic drugs in elderly nursing home residents with and without dementia in Helsinki, Finland. *Drugs and Aging*, 22: 793–800.

Hoti, K., Forman, D. & Hughes, J. (2014). Evaluating an interprofessional disease state and medication management review model. *Journal of Interprofessional Care*, 28: 168–70.

Hoti, K., Hughes, J. & Sunderland, B. (2011). Pharmacy client's attitudes on expanded pharmacist prescribing and the role of agency theory on involved stakeholders. *International Journal of Pharmacy Practice*, 19: 5–12.

Institute for Patient- and Family-Centred Care. (n.d.). Definition of person-centred care. Retrieved 3 August 2014 from http://www.ipfcc.org

Jha, A.K., Orav, E.J., Zheng, J. & Epstein, A.M. (2008). Patients' perception of hospital care in the United States. *New England Journal of Medicine*, 359: 1921–31.

Kitwood, T. (1988). The technical, the personal, and the framing of dementia. *Social Behaviours*, 3: 161–79.

Kitwood, T. (1997). *Dementia reconsidered: The person comes first*. Buckingham, UK: Open University Press.

Knaus, W.A., Draper, E.A., Wagner, D.P. & Zimmerman, J.E. (1986). An evaluation of outcome from intensive care in major medical centres. *Annals of Internal Medicine*, 104: 410–18.

Lane, L. (2000). Client-centred practice: Is it compatible with early discharge hospital-at-home policies? *British Journal of Occupational Therapy*, 63: 310–15.

McDonough, R.P. & Doucette, W.R. (2001). Dynamics of pharmaceutical care: Developing collaborative working relationships between pharmacists and physicians. *Journal of American Pharmaceutical Association*, 41: 682–92.

Mott, D.A., Schommer, J.C., Doucette, W.R. & Kreling, D.H. (1998). Agency theory, drug formularies, and drug product selection: Implications for public policy. *Journal of Public Policy Marketing*, 17: 277–85.

Nair, M. (2006). Nursing management of the patient with Alzheimer's disease. *British Journal of Nursing*, 15: 258–62.

National Institute for Health and Care Excellence (NICE). (2006). Dementia: Supporting people with dementia and their carers in health and social care. *NICE Clinical Guideline*, 42.

Peisah, C. & Skladzien, E. (2014). *The use of restraints and psychotropic medications in people with dementia*. Paper 38. Scullin, ACT: Alzheimer's Australia.

Rogers, C.R. (1961). *On becoming a person*. Boston: Houghton Mifflin.

Royal College of Nursing. (n.d.). Definition of person-centred care. Retrieved 10 August 2014 from http://www.rcn.org.uk

Shaller, D. (2007). *Patient-centred care: What does it take?* New York: The Commonwealth Fund.

Snyder, M.E., Zillich, A.J., Primack, B.A., Rice, K.R., Somma, M.A., Pringle, J.L. & Smith, R.B. (2010). Exploring successful community pharmacist-physician collaborative working relationships using mixed methods. *Administrative Pharmacy*, 6: 307–23.

Steketee, C., Forman, D., Dunston, R., Yassine, T., Matthews, L.R. ... Alliex, S. (2014). Interprofessional health education in Australia: Three research projects informing curriculum renewal and development. *Applied Nursing Research*, 27: 115–20.

Stewart, M., Brown, J.B., Donner, A., McWhinney, I.R., Oates, J., Weston, W.W. & Jordan, J. (2000). The impact of patient-centred care on outcomes. *Journal of Family Practice*, 49: 796–804.

Stone, S. (2008). A retrospective evaluation of the impact of the Planetree patient-centred model of care on inpatient quality outcomes. *Health Environments Research and Design Journal*, July, 1(4): 55–69.

Victorian Government Department of Human Services. (2003). *Improving care for older people: A policy for health services*. Retrieved 7 July 2014 from http://www.health.vic.gov.au

Victorian Government Department of Human Services. (2010). *Person-centred care. Good practice for quality dementia care*. Retrieved 31 March 2015 from http://www.health.vic.gov.au/dementia/images/a2z/checklist31.pdf

Wimo, A. & Prince, M. (2010). *World Alzheimer Report 2010: The global economic impact of dementia*. London: Alzheimer's Disease International.

World Health Organization (WHO). (2000). *The World Health Report 2000 – Health Systems: Improving Performance* (pp. 1–215). Geneva: WHO.

World Health Organization (WHO). (2010). *Patients for patient safety*. Retrieved 12 August 2014 from http://www.who.int

Zillich, A.J., McDonough, R.P., Carter, B.L. & Douchette, W.R. (2004). Influential characteristics of physician/pharmacist collaborative relationships. *Annals of Pharmacotherapy*, 38: 764–70.

9 Understanding ethics and dementia care

Stephan Millett

Learning outcomes

1 Understand the importance of the concepts of self and personhood in the context of dementia.

2 Demonstrate knowledge of ethical concepts.

3 Be able to reflect on the impact that cultural understanding may have on giving or receiving dementia care.

4 Understand that relationships are important in caring for others.

Key terms

- autonomy
- culture
- dementia
- ethics
- palliative care
- value

Introduction

It can be easy to look at ethics as simply following codes or a set of principles that influence what people do. Both of these are important but, in a health setting, particularly one involving dementia care, codes and principles may not be enough because they do not adequately take account of the special situation of someone who needs care, especially those who can be challenging to care for.

Ethics
The body of values and judgements relating to human conduct, especially with respect to the rightness and wrongness of certain actions, and to the motives and ends of such actions.

This chapter discusses some key ethical concepts. It also looks at what might be helpful for carers to understand so they may act ethically towards those with dementia. It shows professionals that **ethics** influences what they do with the information that they have. It is as necessary a part of an interprofessional and evidence-based practice as sound science, good skills or lived experience.

At a basic level, people need to know about ethics simply to get along with each other, as ethics enters into every interaction that they have with others. In some way or other, at its heart, ethical behaviour must take into account how each person might affect others. This means that people should consider the possible consequences of what they do. But ethics is more than thinking about the possible consequences of actions. Each person needs also to reflect on the reasons for doing things, on what sort of person they want to be and how relationships might be valued and nurtured in even the most challenging care environments.

In addition to some of the principles that have become a common element in discussions of ethics, some key concepts and how they work in practice need to be understood. Take trust and promising, for example. Imagine that you ask a friend if you can borrow her car. You promise to bring it back by 5pm, when she needs it to drive home, and you promise to put some fuel in it. You bring it back at 6pm and have not put fuel in it. She has had to miss out on visiting her mum in hospital on the way home and she has to put fuel in herself. A week later, you ask to borrow the car again. She is not keen, but you beg and plead, and she relents. You promise (again) to bring the car back on time and full of fuel. Again you are an hour late and forget to put fuel in. The next time you ask, she says 'No'. You have broken your promises to her, she is not happy with what you have done and she no longer trusts that you will keep your word.

Breaking a promise has consequences. Some consequences are immediate, some are short term, some are delayed and some are long-lasting. At the personal level, breaking a promise may mean that you are not trusted in the future, and may lead to the break-up of friendships and families, or to the loss of jobs and so on. If breaking promises happens on a wider scale, there will be less and less trust between people. This could signal the beginnings of a major breakdown in our relationships, in our communities, in our workplaces and in our society as a whole. One of the reasons this is the case is because, if we are to apply principles, it is important that we all apply sound principles and apply them consistently. Breaking a promise is not a sound principle because if everyone did it then promises would come to have no meaning.

Promising and trust are important, perhaps vitally important, but they are just two of many concepts in ethics. There are also concepts such as fairness, rights, obligations or duties, loyalties, responsibility, care, consequences, virtues and values. Each ethical concept can have an impact on what we do in our working, family and social lives, but this chapter can only touch on some of them.

Ethics and culture

The word 'ethics' comes from the ancient Greek word *ethikos*, which itself comes from the word *ethos*. *Ethos* means something close to custom or habit whereas *ethikos* means to be moral or to show moral character. So, from as far back as early Greece, ethics refers to such things as 'moral character and behaviour' and recognises that behaviour is influenced by the customs or habits of the society or **culture** that we live in. In this way, ethical behaviour is not something that always looks and sounds the same in all societies or cultures. However, although what is right or true in one culture may not be right or true in another, this does not mean that ethics is purely relative to the culture we live in: there are ethical concepts that cultures have in common. In countries that have a Confucian understanding of ethics, respect might be demonstrated through observing *li*, the accepted rituals, customs or etiquette, or by behaving in such a way that *mianzi*, 'face' or reputation, is preserved. In Islam, the concept of *akhlaq* is a disposition that incorporates a requirement for respectful behaviour.

> **Culture**
> The main definition of culture used in this book is: 'Culture is all aspects of life, the totality of meanings, ideas and beliefs shared by individuals within a group of people. Culture is learned, it includes language, values, norms, customs.' (http://www.design.iastate.edu/NAB/about/thinkingskills/cultural_context/cultural.html).

To take another example, most cultures have a concept of murder, but there may be differences in what is regarded as murder. In a particular society, it may not be considered murder if a member of one clan kills a member of another clan, but killing a member of your own clan – without going through some process of justice – would be murder. On a more everyday level, all cultures have a concept of showing respect but it may look and sound different between cultures. For example, in many Islamic societies showing the soles of your feet is considered rude or disrespectful and in many Australian indigenous communities direct eye contact may be considered a sign of disrespect.

What counts as respectful behaviour differs between cultures, and, when we encounter people from other cultures, we may cause offence without meaning to unless we take the time to find out how it is polite and correct to behave among them.

There can be much that is lost in translation between cultures: not just the translation of words, but also of actions. Every time we attempt to translate meaning from one culture to our own there is a degree of mistranslation and, as a result, we do not understand things exactly the way they are understood in the other culture. It is important to try hard to understand. This can be done by focusing on the following:

1 the actual words used or the actions observed;

2 what we understand from the words or actions;

3 then to ask what might be meant by them, what might the speaker have intended?

Here it is important to note that although something might be seen as a criticism or an insult it may not be meant that way: it may be misinterpreted. The first need is to *understand* what is meant, and why. However, it is important to remember that understanding is not the same as agreeing. It is possible to understand another person's position without agreeing with it.

Special demands and challenges to traditional ethics

Dementia presents ethical challenges for carers. It also presents challenges to the principles that underpin Western health ethics. The most widely used of these principles are set out in Beauchamp and Childress (2009) and form the core of biomedical ethics. They are:

Dementia
Dementia is now referred to as a neurocognitive disorder (NCD) (American Psychiatric Association, 2013), that is, the result of chronic or progressive damage to the brain.

- respect for persons (or autonomy);
- bringing a benefit, not causing harm;
- justice (who gets what).

However, despite their widespread use and undoubted power in environments such as research ethics and some clinical environments, they are not necessarily the best tools to use in addressing ethics in dementia care. There are challenges facing the effective use of these principles – challenges that are made more difficult to address if people with dementia continue to be regarded in terms of persons who are in the process of losing their minds or their self – so an alternative way of thinking about the ideas of self and person is also needed. This alternative way of thinking is discussed later in the chapter but before considering this it is important to understand that a person requires respect.

Respect for persons

Autonomy, agency and respect

When looking at the major principles of bioethics, it is usual to begin with the idea of respecting persons for what they are in themselves and not for some other purpose; an idea most closely associated with philosophical thinking adapted from the work of Immanuel Kant (1724–1804). In adopting this idea, people are to be considered valuable for their own sake and not mere 'things' that can be used for someone else's benefit.

In modern ethics, respect for persons is often interpreted as respect for an individual's **autonomy** – usually understood as the capacity to make rational uncoerced and informed decisions about the things that affect their life. This is coupled to the concept of *agency* – the capacity that humans and many other living things have to affect the world in some way. Agency in humans is often viewed as something that we have some control over. This includes what is known as goal-directed agency, such as making a decision and

> **Autonomy**
> The capacity to make rational, uncoerced and informed decisions about the things that affect one's life.

acting on it. In health care environments, respect for a person's autonomy usually comes down to making sure that each person actively consents to a procedure or action.

This sounds reasonably simple until we start to look more closely and understand that to be able to *consent* we must be able to *understand* what is involved in a procedure or an action. This is hard enough for mature, competent adults faced with having to make a decision, especially when they are under stress, or when the information is provided in technical language, or given in language that reduces complex issues and risks to a level that is too simple. But what happens when the people whom we are caring for are becoming less able to understand information, less able to make what we think are rational decisions and less able to act on their decisions? The first consideration is that being *less able* does not mean they are *not able* to make decisions. It is not a case of either being able or not able – there are shades of grey – and an approach to ethics based on respecting autonomy does not deal well with situations where rationality is not clearly present. There are also other ways in which placing an emphasis on rationality is a problem.

People who are gradually losing their abilities to reason and to act on reasoned choices are frequently regarded as, in some way, losing their self or becoming less of a person (Allen & Coleman, 2006; Cohen & Eisdorfer, 2002; Davis, 2004; MacRae, 2010). In an approach to ethics based on decisions by rational autonomous persons, it is too easy to move into a way of thinking where the obligation of a professional to protect vulnerable people overrides the very autonomy that is so important to our understanding of what a person is. There is a tendency to take over and, paternalistically, to give people what professionals think they need rather than continue to work with them to find out what their needs are.

A dilemma of personhood

The perception that people with dementia suffer a loss of self has wide currency and informs quite a lot of both lay and professional understanding of the disease. However, the idea that people with dementia are losing their 'self', or that they are not the same person as they were, presents a clear dilemma: a choice between two approaches, neither of which is desirable.

If a view is taken that people with dementia are in the process of losing their 'self', the end result of the process of loss is that the individual is thought to have no 'self' and comes to be regarded as no longer a person. If the end result is someone who is not autonomous, is not rational and has limited agency – in effect, a non-person – and an approach to ethics based on respect for *persons* is taken then there is a danger of moving people with dementia into a category where they are thought not to have the same rights as others and where, as a consequence, it is easy to think that professional carers do not have the same obligations to them as they do to other people.

If a view is taken that people with dementia continue to have or continue to be a 'self' throughout their life, there is a risk of putting an unreasonable burden on family carers. The burden might include:

- People are denied a proper mourning for the loss of their loved one as the dementia progresses.
- Carers may feel guilt or shame at their changed feelings towards the obviously changing 'person'.
- Carers effectively become caught up in defining those they care for as disabled and as having a progressive deficit. The story becomes one of loss.

One of the ways to resolve a dilemma, such as that just outlined, is to identify and challenge the assumptions on which it is based. Here, a major assumption is that we have **value** because we are selves, or persons. But, there is no widespread agreement on what a 'self' is and what its loss might constitute. Either there needs to be agreement on what a 'person' or 'self' is – for example, something that is rational, aware that it exists, able to communicate, able to plan for the future and able to act on those plans – or another source of value needs to be found.

> **Value**
> The regard that something is held to deserve; the importance, worth or usefulness of something.

Loss of self is most commonly seen as a symptom of reducing cognitive capacity. Cognitive capacity does diminish progressively in people with dementia because that is one of the defining characteristics. However, does cognitive capacity affect the *value* of an individual and, if so, how? By using cognitive capacity and the ability to reason as determinants of value, there is a risk of denying relevance to emotion, embodiment and a changing inner life as well as, at a fundamental level, to existence itself.

An additional problem is that of distinguishing the symptoms of dementia from what is normal. Hughes, for example, says that 'at the most objective end of "mental" illness (that is, in the field of "organic" dementias) ... there is no hard scientific boundary between disease and normality' (Hughes, Louw & Sabat, 2006, p. 2). If the difference between what is normal and what is a case of organic dementia isn't easily known, how can value judgements be made about people based on whether they are one or the other – normal or having dementia?

Bringing a benefit and not causing harm

Dementia also presents a challenge for the linked concepts of happiness, benefit and harm.

Happiness is generally thought to be desirable: the more that people are happy, the better things are. Under the Greatest Happiness Principle, the most ethical way to act is in such a way that our actions bring about the greatest happiness for the greatest number of those affected (Mill, 1860). This consequentialist approach has the great advantage that it is common sense to try to maximise benefits and minimise harms. It has the great disadvantages that we cannot know in advance that our actions will bring benefit or harm and that we cannot measure happiness very well.

The Greatest Happiness Principle is commonly linked with what is known as the Harm Principle, which states that 'the only purpose for which power can be rightfully exercised over any member of a civilised community, against his will, is to prevent harm to others' (Mill, 1860, pp. 21–2).

These two principles can be looked at along with the question of *restraint* for people with dementia. Restraint takes many forms, from locked doors in care facilities, to electronic tags, to physical restraints and chemical restraints – pharmaceuticals. Often the justification is to protect people from self-inflicted harm but, following the Harm Principle set out by Mill, the only justified reason is to prevent harm to others. However, not all restraints are put in place to protect others. And the idea that the community has a responsibility to protect people from themselves is highly controversial. If we really took this idea to heart, where would it end? No one would be allowed to drink alcohol, drive cars, smoke cigarettes or do extreme sports because they all are highly likely to cause harm to those doing these things.

If putting people with dementia in secure care, with or without other restraints, is thought of in terms of the Greatest Happiness Principle, it could be argued that the general community is better off – is happier – by not having to deal with increasing numbers of people with dementia of varying severity. This has to be weighed against the possible harms or benefits to people with dementia – but that is not so easy to do either. If the projected increased happiness of the general community is thought to outweigh the cost or harm to the people placed in secure care, then the Greatest Happiness Principle would justify restraining people with dementia. But how can happiness be measured? To be clear, the happiness being discussed is really better thought of as 'well-being'. It is not the sort of momentary joy someone might get from winning a raffle or getting good news about a medical test. Even so, how can it be measured? Can the total benefit to the community, in having people with dementia restrained, outweigh the negative effects on well-being from restraining them? The simple answer is that it can't.

The Greatest Happiness Principle underpins the approach to ethics called 'utilitarianism', a variety of consequentialism, where the consequences of a decision or action are taken to be the most relevant consideration. One of the most commonly voiced types of utilitarianism is 'preference utilitarianism', where the satisfaction of a person's preferences – what is in their best interests – is the key to their well-being. But how do health professionals ensure that they are fully aware of the preferences of people with dementia and whether those preferences should be met, given that many people simply do not always know what is in their best interests? How do people with dementia ensure that their preferences are satisfied when their agency, their ability to act, is declining and the structures of care increasingly take power away from them? How do professionals ensure that preferences are addressed when every person's experience of satisfaction is unique? And how do they overcome the prejudice that preference utilitarianism has in favour of rational, autonomous agents – people who can make the sorts of preference choices required?

These are difficult questions. The main point of asking them here is to highlight that, as long as primary consideration is given to the idea of a person who is a rational, autonomous agent, professionals will struggle to address adequately the ethical issues in dementia care.

Justice

The final concept in Beauchamp and Childress's list of principles is justice. This is a highly important concept in ethics but it is also a hugely difficult concept to understand. The idea goes back at least to Plato and his book *The Republic*. Although there are many ways to think about justice, in health ethics the concept is commonly concentrated on distributive justice: who gets what and when they should get it. It is a major feature of health policy and politics.

From a policy perspective professionals might ask whether funding for aged care should be increased as the population ages. And, similarly, whether funding for dementia care should be increased as the numbers of people with dementia increase. The money available is limited, so to provide more funding, more money needs to be found from somewhere. Usually this means reducing money spent on something else – but what should be cut to pay for aged care and dementia care, and on what basis should the decision be made? What principles should guide this decision?

One approach to justice involves a thought experiment called the 'veil of ignorance' (Rawls, 1971, pp. 136–42), where we imagine that we are behind a curtain or veil and have to come up with principles that our community or society should operate by. When the veil is taken away we take up roles in the community. But before the veil is removed we do not know if we will be male or female, young or old, qualified or unqualified, well or unwell, cognitively sound or cognitively impaired, English speaking or non-English speaking, African or European and so on. When the veil is taken away, and those affected have to take up roles that they did not choose, they have to be satisfied with the principles under which they have chosen their society to operate. This applies whether they find themselves as a day labourer, a homeless person with dementia or a neurosurgeon. If a principle of survival of the fittest is chosen, will they be satisfied when they find out they are old and losing their memory? If a principle of individual responsibility and user pays is selected, will they be satisfied if they are single, sick and without assets? If a principle that the government should pay is favoured, will they be happy to pay the taxes?

So, what principles should be adopted to ensure that people live in a just society with a just solution to the problems that aged care and dementia care present? There is no easy answer and some of the key principles of ethics, when applied to dementia, do not really help to resolve the problem. However, one area – the ethics of care (Gilligan, 1982; Held, 2006; Noddings, 2002) – offers some hope because it does not focus on rules and rational judgement alone, but recognises that emotional attachment and relationships are also highly important. Before looking at ethics of care more closely, it is important to address in more detail what a person is.

Self and personhood

Since at least the influential work of Tom Kitwood (1997), person-centred care has been significantly important for those working in dementia care. However, a number of ethical issues with dementia relate to the idea that those with dementia are in a process of losing their 'self', something that Herskovits (1995) says is implied in the very idea of Alzheimer's disease. For Davis (2004), Kitwood's attempt to preserve a sense of personhood – or 'persons-without-awareness' – in people with dementia can damage or delegitimise the feelings of carers, who do not recognise any semblance of the relationship they used to have with the one they are caring for. The perception of loss of self presents a problem for the welfare of people with dementia as it can lead to depersonalised treatment (Ashworth & Ashworth, 2003; Kontos & Naglie, 2006; Millett, 2011) and possibly abuse.

However, there is confusion about the meanings of the terms 'self', 'selfhood' and 'personhood', and they are often used interchangeably. While questioning what a *self* is may seem to be an abstract activity, it does relate to problems of practical importance. One is the problem of what is in the best interests of people with dementia. An interest is a capacity to be harmed or benefited, and inflicting harm is a violation of an interest (Feinberg, 1973, p. 26). But do we try to satisfy the preference interests of someone – what they want to do – or their welfare interests? Welfare interests are also known as vital interests. They are basic interests because if they are not satisfied we will suffer and may even die. This makes them more morally relevant than other interests.

When questioning what is meant by the terms 'self' and 'person', it is pertinent to ask whether having any special cognitive property, such as being self-aware, brings a special moral status. If it doesn't, as for example Tom Beauchamp (1999) argues, there is a need to look beyond the idea of a 'self' or 'person' for the source of moral value.

To understand the problem of the idea of a self, the Scottish philosopher David Hume is a good place to start. Hume ([1739] 1978) argued that people do not have any idea of '*self*, ...' (p. 251) but rather 'are nothing but a bundle or collection of different perceptions' (p. 252) and their minds are 'a kind of theatre, where several perceptions successively make their appearance' and which have 'no *simplicity* ... at one time, nor *identity* in different' (p. 253). That is, a self is not one single thing and is not the same right now as it was a year ago or will be in a year's time. Hume (1978, p. 252) also considered *perception* to be fundamental:

> For my part, when I enter most intimately into what I call myself, I always stumble on some particular perception or other, of heat or cold, light or shade, love or hatred, pain or pleasure. I never can catch myself at any time without a perception, and never can observe any thing but the perception.

Perception may be fundamental, but there almost certainly has to be a 'body' to do the perceiving and, in the philosophical literature about dementia, there has been an increasing focus on the idea of embodiment: the idea that people are fundamentally physical bodies and engage with and make sense of the world because of and through their bodies. A useful discussion of embodiment and self in dementia, which focuses on the importance of perception, is Kontos' (2004, 2005) Model of Embodied Selfhood that she described as a mix of primordial and socio-cultural characteristics of the pre-reflective body; that is, the body and how it fits into the social world, *before* a person starts to think about it.

But even if selfhood is a mix of primordial and social characteristics, has this advanced the discussion? This approach does not address adequately the effect on all involved of believing there is a loss of self.

Given the complexities in the ideas of selfhood and personhood, and the widespread misunderstanding of them, should notions of self and personhood be left aside to focus on the continuity, over time, of an embodied individual and people's attitude to that individual? Should professionals concentrate on the various ways that people with dementia are *present* rather than *absent*?

Valuing

One way to view people in terms of how they are *present* is to view the life of people with dementia as one of inner change rather than as a process of increasing loss. Once a move is made away from the idea that dementia involves only disease and loss, as does Davis (2004) for example, it becomes possible for carers to change the way that they interact with those with dementia. Rethinking the way that people with dementia engage with their world also requires others to rethink their own engagement with their world and with the ethics of caring for those with dementia.

Put aside the notions of self and personhood for the moment, and focus on the idea that when a profession is faced with an individual who has dementia it is seeing a being with an inner life, a being with value simply because he or she has a 'life-world' – a constructed, meaning-full world revealed to him or her through the senses.

Using a concept of 'life-world' offers a useful way to understand the importance of embodiment and individuality to the world of those with dementia. It is a way that does not rely on a notion of 'self' or of 'person' and so does not get caught up in ideas like 'loss of self' or an individual being a 'different person'.

If it is understood that all organisms, including all humans, use their senses to build a unique view of the world, then a view of dementia can be developed in which those with the disease –even with very late stage dementia – can be recognised as continuing to have an inner life and continue to both experience and communicate with the world around them (Millett, 2011). This experience may look, sound and feel different to their experience of the world before dementia, and it may not be understood, but it is, nonetheless, their experience, and is to be valued and respected.

Everyone receives information from the surrounding environment through sense organs. This allows each individual to create, from the information received through the body, a 'world' that has meaning unique to that individual. We each receive and interpret signs from the world around us. These can be the sounds of music, the touch of a friend, the smell of food, the sight of a sunset, words or all of these in some way together.

People with dementia continue to receive inputs through their senses. They continue to be complex beings who make sense of the world by interpreting signs. And they continue to have a unique value even though the way that they receive, interpret and make meaning of signs is changing. This unique value is sometimes called 'intrinsic' or 'inherent value'.

The point of talking about the way individuals use their senses to create a world is to show that there is a way to value people that does not rely on the idea of a self or of a person. People interact with their world, they make sense of their world in their own way and they occupy a unique place in the world. All of this gives them a unique value that is independent of whether they can remember things or understand clearly.

There is a directly experienced world for people with dementia, even in the presence of severe cognitive degradation. For example, it is clear that people with even advanced dementia can feel pain and that they can have an *affective* response to certain stimuli: they can laugh, cry, get frustrated, get angry and so on. An affective or emotional response – signs of happiness, sadness, frustration, anger and the like – indicates that there is an interior life even if it isn't fully understood. From the affective responses it can be seen that people with even late-stage dementia still react to, engage with and co-create a directly experienced world. People with dementia still experience a world and have an inner life, but how might knowing this change the way people feel towards them and act towards them?

If carers can be helped to let go of the idea of the 'person' with dementia as an individual in decay, they may be able to understand that the one being cared for is, in effect, continuing the process of creating his or her own unique sense of the world through the changed perceptions that come with dementia. If carers can do this then they may be better able to recognise that the individual with dementia continues to have value and is someone to whom they have an obligation. Family carers, who let go of the idea of an individual in decay, may also be able to manage a 'guiltless grieving' (Davis, 2004) while continuing to provide respectful care.

By moving to a position that doesn't rely on a notion of self, what attitude might professionals take to those with dementia, most particularly advanced dementia? One strong candidate is a special way of understanding sympathy as:

> a feeling or emotion that (a) responds to some apparent threat or obstacle to an individual's good or well-being, (b) has that individual himself as object, and (c) involves concern for him, and thus for his well-being, *for his sake.* (Darwall, 1998, p. 261)

Sympathy in this sense has nothing to do with pity and it is not the same as empathy, which is understanding or feeling what something might be like for others. And it is not a token show of emotion. It is always felt from the perspective of the one who is caring. It is a form of genuinely caring *for* someone for the sake *of* that someone. If Darwall's special notion of sympathy is adopted, carers will care *for* those with dementia and do what is in their best interests, *because* it is best for them and not because the rules say so or it fits with what carers want to do.

This can be related to one of the defining elements of the professions – that the professional has a moral fiduciary obligation to their client or patient.

The professions differ from other occupations in that it is widely thought that members of professions need to meet the following criteria:

- They need to have spent years, usually at a university, learning a large body of formal knowledge.
- They need to put that body of knowledge to work in the service of a client or patient.
- Their right to practise what they have learned is controlled in some way by a self-regulating body of peers, such as a medical college for specialist physicians.
- They are generally required to undergo continuing professional development throughout their careers.
- They need to have an ethical focus.

For Robert Sokolowski (1991), this ethical focus is a relationship where:

> The exercise of professional judgment and skill must, first of all, be for the client's good. This obligation does not stem from any personal benevolence or private virtue on the part of the professional, but from the very nature of the relationship between professional and client [p. 28] … The relationship between professional and client is a fiduciary relationship. The client trusts the professional and entrusts him or herself – not just his or her possessions – to the professional [p. 31].

The fiduciary relationship is a relationship of trust. The client or patient has to trust (in some way) the professional – and the professional has to make sure that this trust is warranted by acting in the best interests of the client. This goes beyond merely doing what the patient or client wants as they are seldom in a position to know what the options are or how best to weigh one option against another. Clients need advice or treatment from professionals but they have to make themselves vulnerable to the professional before they can get help (a nurse may need a patient to undress, a doctor will need highly personal information and so on). Patients or clients are vulnerable to the power that professionals have but they must trust the professionals in order to get help from them. Professionals, on the other hand, have moral obligations to nurture and protect the trust that patients or clients must place in them. That obligation is a moral fiduciary obligation.

I-Thou and care

Despite the criticisms of his focus on person-centredness in dementia care, Kitwood's (1997) insight on this and the practices that flow from it are still vitally important. To understand Kitwood's position, we need to understand that it is founded on Buber's 'I Thou relationship' (1923; 1937).This relationship has three components, an 'I', a 'Thou' and a 'Between'. That is, it involves two individuals and something that exists between them. Everyone reading this is an 'I' because you can say 'I did this ... I want ...' etc. Every one of us can also be a 'thou' in the eyes of another. It may be worth explaining this word a little because it is an old word that does not get used much anymore. In English, the word 'thou' has been overtaken by the word 'you'. But the word 'you' can refer to an individual or to a group. When a friend comes to visit she might be asked: 'Would you like a cup of tea?' This use of 'you' could be replaced with 'thou'. (In old language we might ask: 'Wouldst thou partake of tea?'). In grammatical terms, 'thou' is an old version of the second person singular. If we said 'Wouldst thou partake of tea?' it could only refer to one individual at a time (usually the one we are looking at). If I were to use colloquial Australian words to ask a group whether they wanted tea, I might say 'Would youse like a cup of tea?' Americans might say 'you all' (y'all). So, there is an I and a Thou, but these cannot really be separated because they depend on each other. For there to be any sort of social interaction, there needs always to be at least an I and a Thou, and the relationship between them. This relationship is, for Allen and Coleman (2006, p. 210), one of 'subject to subject, of self-disclosure and intimacy', which can 'fall away into subject-object, I-It, that is, coolness and detachment' when caring for someone with dementia. For this reason, the Between is important.

The I-Thou is intentionally hyphenated, and we might think of the Between as the 'hyphen-zone', the place and the space that is between an I and a Thou, between me and you. It is always there whenever an I and a Thou meet. In addition to Buber, the work of Levinas (1981) delves deeply into the I and Thou and, for him, each human addresses an ought-to-care to each other human (Krueger, 2008). That is, every human has an obligation to other humans, an obligation that takes on particular force when we come face to face with another human. When we see the face of another, Levinas says, we are *called* to care. So, we might also think of the hyphen-zone in the 'I-Thou' as the zone of care. It is always there, so we always have an obligation to care.

The ethics of care can be seen as fundamentally relational – it always takes account of the relationship between an I and a Thou – and involves caring about and caring for (Noddings, 2002). If I care *about* a matter then it is on my moral radar, it is a matter of ethical importance, even if I cannot act to fix the problem. If I care *for* someone then I am actively doing something that is in their interests. To caring about and caring for, 'taking care' might also be added, which is attention to detail, doing your job properly and watching out for problems. The ethics of care is fundamentally relational, and for Gilligan (1982, p. 19) it is also something in which:

> the moral problem arises from conflicting responsibilities rather than from competing rights and requires for its resolution a mode of thinking that is contextual and narrative rather than formal and abstract. This conception of morality as concerned with the activity of care centres moral development around the understanding of responsibility and relationships …

If moral development requires understanding of responsibility and relationships, then carers wishing to behave ethically need to recognise that they have obligations to those with dementia and to remember that these people are still members of communities and families (Racher, 2007), and that they have value because of that. However, at a fundamental level, people with dementia are still 'the subject of a life' that is continuing and has value in and of itself, whether others can 'get through to them' or not.

There is much more that may be said on the ethics of care, as a theory, but the takeaway message is that it fundamentally focuses on responsibilities and relationships in preference to recognising rights and following rules. Perhaps the essence of care is in the hyphen-zone: people are born with an obligation to others and when they come to face another they have an obligation to ask: 'How can I help you?' even if those they are asking cannot answer. The role of carers is to find the best way to work out what the needs of the clients are and to act in their interests, for their sake.

Carers, care for yourself too

Another aspect of care ethics is that carers have an obligation to care for themselves. Burnout from caring too much is a very real possibility in carers, especially among **palliative care** and hospice workers who, to avoid burnout, 'need to develop a plan of self-care to successfully balance their own needs with the needs of their patients' (Hill Jones, 2005, pp. 125–6). To do this they need first to reflect on their own motivation and move to a mature understanding of it by tapping into a bigger picture of their calling. Following this, the care plan needs to deal with four areas of well-being: physical; emotional/cognitive; relational; and spiritual (Hill Jones, 2005).

Of particular use in avoiding burnout is Purtilo's (2005) approach to ethical decision making, which recognises that ethical problems can arise through ethical distress, ethical dilemmas or from what she calls the locus of authority problem, as follows:

> **Palliative care**
> Palliative care is an approach that improves the quality of life of patients and their families facing the problems associated with life-threatening illness, through the prevention and relief of suffering by means of early identification and impeccable assessment and treatment of pain and other problems: physical, psychosocial and spiritual.

- Ethical distress can stop people from acting. This can be a barrier preventing them from doing what they know is right or a barrier that comes about because they know something is wrong, but are not sure exactly what it is.
- If a person faces an ethical dilemma, they have two or more courses of action open to them, but they cannot choose both and, whichever course they choose, someone will suffer. Dilemmas can arise because of a conflict in such things as loyalties, principles or values.
- The locus of authority problem is the problem of knowing who has or should have the authority to make an important ethical decision. Professionals can reduce their ethical distress if they understand that there are ethical issues they do not have the authority to fix, and so cannot fix, and should refer the issue to someone who has the authority to fix the problem.

Professionals should use the Ethics First Aid© checklist, in Figure 9.1, when they are facing a situation that they think may be an ethical issue.

Conclusion

Ethics, at its most fundamental, requires those making decisions to have regard for others, but when the other is a person living with dementia – someone who is 'deeply forgetful' (Post 2006) – it can be difficult to apply some of the common principles of bioethics. Dementia challenges traditional approaches to bioethical engagement because it can undermine the sense that people are dealing with a person who is a source of value.

> ## Ethics First Aid©
>
> **Have you listened carefully enough to understand the problem?**
>
> **Do you have the information you need?**
>
> **What sort of problem is it?**
>
> - **Conflict of interest?** Have you addressed it in a transparent way?
> - **Communication?** Can you help others to understand the problem and find solutions?
> - **Dilemma?** Have you sought help?
> - **Locus of authority?** If you can't address the problem, have you passed it on to the person who has the authority or responsibility to fix it?
>
> **Principles**
>
> - Are you minimising harm?
> - Have you considered the consequences to all those affected? Now? In the future?
> - Are you being guided by a sound principle that you would want others to use?
> - Are you acting in a way that maintains strong and healthy relationships?
>
> **Are you being true to your values?**

FIGURE 9.1   *Ethics First Aid© checklist*
Reproduced with permission from Stephan Millett

Finding an alternative approach to ethical engagement with those who are deeply forgetful requires carers to acknowledge that the individual's life continues, that he or she continues to be the subject of a narrative, continue to have an inner life and continue to have unique value. There is also a need to understand that, although the deeply forgetful may also have fewer preference interests than they once had, they continue to have welfare interests that carers are under an obligation to ensure are satisfied. How this obligation is honoured will vary with every individual cared for, but there are common elements underlying ethical engagement in every case. Harm needs to be minimised. There is a need to consider the consequences of actions for all those affected. Carers need to ensure that the principles they employ are ones that they would want others to use on themselves in similar circumstances. They also need to act in ways that help maintain relationships between the person with dementia and their families, their carers and others who work with, live with or are otherwise affected by them.

Caring for people with dementia can be challenging, not least because the ethical challenges are significant. Understanding ethical obligations, understanding the types of ethical problems that might be encountered and understanding how those problems might best be addressed may help professionals and other carers to care better for those people who depend deeply on the quality of care they receive. But in order to care for others, carers must also care for themselves.

Self-directed learning activities

In this chapter, the self-directed learning activities are based around the case study and are therefore together in this section.

Omar's story

Case study

Omar Masoor is in his late 70s and lives with his 50-year-old daughter, Ameena, and her family. Ameena is married to Khaleel and they have three daughters, with 17-year-old Haniya being the only one still at home.

Omar is a Shia Muslim originally from Iran. His wife died five years ago and since then he has lived with Ameena. He has been diagnosed with dementia and, in recent months, has had increasing incidents where he has lost bowel and bladder control. Ameena and Khaleel are struggling to cope. Both are well-educated and, having lived in Australia for more than 20 years, speak very good English. Khaleel works as an engineer and Ameena is a primary school teacher. Both are professed Muslims, but this is not obvious from the way they dress and how they live.

Omar has periods where he understands well what is going on but increasingly he forgets what has been told to him. He speaks Farsi and has basic English. In recent months, however, he appears not to understand English and increasingly he will only respond to Farsi. Ameena and Khaleel both speak Farsi well and can communicate about daily living with Omar. Haniya has limited Farsi. She feels conflicted about her grandfather living with the family: she values her grandfather but sometimes has had to deal personally with his incontinence and his wandering. It bothers her also that sometimes her grandfather seems to look through her as if she is not there and sometimes seems not to know who she is.

Ameena and Khaleel decide that they need to get some daytime help for Omar so that he can stay in their home. They want Omar to be part of the decision making. The couple seek advice from a dementia care not-for-profit organisation. They take Omar to meet Sharon, a second-generation Australian native English speaker, whose job is to conduct a needs analysis for each potential client of her organisation. Sharon is in her 30s, has two children and lives in a house she is buying with her partner. Her maternal grandmother in England died recently, having lived with dementia for several years.

If possible, discuss in small groups:

1 What information might Sharon need that could help her identify the needs of the family?

2 To what extent, and how, should Sharon take into account each of the people in the household who have an interest in what happens with Omar?

3 What might be some of the issues that the family could face in the coming months and years that are:
   a related to dementia, specifically
   b related to the cultural needs of Omar, Khaleel and Ameena?

4 Using the facts in this case study, identify issues that the family must face now and in the not-too-distant future. Imagine you are Khaleel and Ameena.
   a What values are you likely to emphasise in making decisions? (A value is something that guides you in the way you live your life.)
   b What principles or other ethical concepts might you emphasise in coming to a decision about what you might do with Omar?
   c What loyalties might influence you?
   d What assumptions are you making? Have you carried any preconceptions into your understanding of the family and their situation?

5 To whom or what do the people involved have an obligation and what is the nature of the obligation? For each person, make a chart like the one below (Figure 9.2) and fill it in.

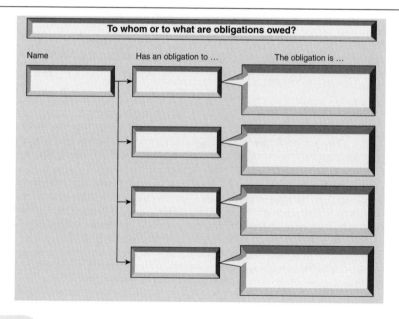

To whom or to what are obligations owed?

Name   Has an obligation to ...   The obligation is ...

FIGURE
9.2   *To be or not to be*

Omar's mental state declines. The family have looked after him at home, but Haniya spends most of her time with her sister and brother-in-law. Omar is bed-bound, incontinent and largely unresponsive. For complex reasons, Khaleel and Ameena feel that they should keep Omar with them.

Reflective questions

1 What might be some of the ethical issues in this situation?
2 What might be some of the consequences for each person: now, soon and in the future?
3 What principle would you want to apply here if you thought you might be in the same situation as any of the people in the story?
4 What relationships should be taken into account, and how?
5 Is the situation fair to Haniya and her sister?

Omar gave no advance directive as to how he wanted to be cared for.

1 How might you, as the coordinator of Omar's care, advise Khaleel and Ameena? Take into account their loyalties, obligations and cultural values (as you understand them).

2 What might be the consequences for all concerned?

3 What principle might apply that you would want all others to apply if you were Omar, Khaleel and Ameena?

4 What relationships are still important and why?

The story of Ms T

Case study

Ms T's husband had been dead 10 years when she was diagnosed with probable Alzheimer's and placed in a nursing home. She is prone to wandering and one night came to the room of a younger cognitively impaired man. A nurse found them both naked in bed. Ms T was weeping. The next day, Ms T's daughter-in-law said that Ms T told her about the incident and that she was still upset. Ms T was unwilling to tell her son directly as she was afraid he would get angry. The son brought a law suit for negligence against the nursing home.

In the court case, the lawyer for the nursing home said that, although Ms T was 'briefly' upset about what the daughter-in-law had said was a violation, she soon forgot about the incident. Therefore, the defence argued that she had not experienced significant 'lasting' harm and thus the case was frivolous. The lawyer called into question whether Ms T did in fact express her grief and whether, at her stage of dementia, she really could have an authentic understanding of what had happened.

(based on a case in Post, 2006)

Reflective questions

1 What harm might Ms T have suffered from the event described above?
   - In addressing this, ask yourself whether it is clear what has happened. Has a wrong been done?
2 Should any possible harm be taken seriously here?
   - In deciding whether an event is harmful, why might it matter that a person no longer remembers a situation which, at the time, was likely to be traumatic?
3 Would your answer be different if you were asked to comment on a young person who suffers amnesia related to post-traumatic stress following an assault?

Follow-up

In his original version of the above scenario, Post (2006) argued that the first harm was to Ms T's remaining self-identity (for he believed that she still had core values that had informed her life to this point, and there were periods of insight). He noted that we should work to create an environment in which Ms T's connections with the past are cultivated in order to enhance her sense of security and well-being. The second harm to Ms T was an emotional harm, as emotional life should be especially respected, even if emotional upset is apparently relatively short-lived.

The fact that Ms T was deeply forgetful was not enough to prevent her from harm or enough to have her to be regarded as being less worthy of moral consideration than others. Being rational is not, in itself, enough as a basis for moral consideration; otherwise newborns would not be morally considerable.

References

Allen, F.B. & Coleman, P.G. (2006). Spiritual perspectives on the person with dementia: Identity and personhood. In J.C. Hughes, S.J. Louw & S.R. Sabat (eds) *Dementia: Mind meaning and the person*. Oxford: Oxford University Press.

Ashworth, A. & Ashworth, P. (2003). The lifeworld as phenomenon and as research heuristic, exemplified by a study of the lifeworld of a person suffering Alzheimer's disease. *Journal of Phenomenological Psychology*, 34(2): 179–205.

Beauchamp, T. (1999). The failure of theories of personhood. *Kennedy Institute of Ethics Journal*, 9(4): 309–24.

Beauchamp, T. & Childress, J. (2009). *Principles of biomedical ethics* (6th edn). Oxford: Oxford University Press.

Buber, M. (1923; 1937). *I and thou* (R.G. Smith, trans.). Edinburgh: T. & T. Clark.

Cohen, D. & Eisdorfer, C. (2002). *The loss of self: A family resource for the care of Alzheimer's disease.* New York: W.W. Norton.

Darwall, S. (1998). Empathy, sympathy, care. *Philosophical Studies,* 89: 261–82.

Davis, D.H.J. (2004). Dementia: Sociological and philosophical constructions. *Social Science and Medicine,* 58: 369–78.

Feinberg, J. (1973). *Social philosophy.* Englewood Cliffs, NJ: Prentice Hall.

Gilligan, C. (1982). *In a different voice: Psychological theory and women's development.* Cambridge, MA: Harvard University Press.

Held, V. (2006). *The ethics of care: Personal, political, and global.* New York: Oxford University Press.

Herskovits, E. (1995). Struggling over subjectivity: Debates about the 'self' and Alzheimer's disease. *Medical Anthropology Quarterly,* June, 9(2): 146–64.

Hill Jones, S. (2005). A self-care for hospice workers. *American Journal of Hospice and Palliative Medicine,* March/April, 22(2).

Hughes, J.C., Louw, S.J. & Sabat, S.R. (2006). Seeing whole. In J.C. Hughes, S.J. Louw & S.R. Sabat (eds) *Dementia: Mind, meaning, and the person.* Oxford: Oxford University Press.

Hume, D. (1978). *A treatise of human nature* (2nd edn). Oxford: Clarendon Press.

Kitwood, T.M. (1997). *Dementia reconsidered: The person comes first.* Buckingham, UK: Open University Press.

Kontos, P.C. (2004). Ethnographic reflections on selfhood, embodiment and Alzheimer's disease. *Ageing and Society,* 24(06): 829–49. doi: 10.1017/S0144686X04002375

Kontos, P.C. (2005). Embodied selfhood in Alzheimer's disease: Rethinking person-centred care. *Dementia,* 4(4): 553.

Kontos, P.C. & Naglie, G. (2006). Expressions of personhood in Alzheimer's: Moving from ethnographic text to performing ethnography. *Qualitative Research,* 6: 301.

Krueger, J.W. (2008). Levinasian reflections on somaticity and the ethical self. *Inquiry,* 51(6): 603–26.

Levinas, E. (1981). *Otherwise than being* (A. Lingis, trans.). Pittsburgh, PA: Duquesne University Press.

MacRae, R. (2010). Managing identity while living with Alzheimer's disease. *Qualitative Health Research,* 20(3): 293–305.

Mill, J.S. (1860). *On liberty,* Vol. 25. Harvard Classics. Retrieved from http://www.constitution.org/jsm/liberty.htm

Millett, S. (2011). Self and embodiment: A bio-phenomenological approach to dementia. *Dementia,* 10(4): 509–22. doi: 10.1177/1471301211409374

Noddings, N. (2002). *Educating moral people: A caring alternative to character education.* Williston, VT: Teachers College Press.

Post, S.G. (2006). Respectare: Moral respect for the lives of the deeply forgetful. In J.C. Hughes, S.J. Louw & S.R. Sabat (eds) *Dementia: Mind, meaning, and the person*. Oxford: Oxford University Press.

Purtilo, R. (2005). *Ethical dimensions in the health professions*. Philadelphia: Elsevier-Saunders.

Racher, F.E. (2007). The evolution of ethics for community practice. *Journal of Community Health Nursing*, Spring, 24(1): 65–76.

Rawls, J. (1971). *A theory of justice*. Cambridge, MA.: Belknap Harvard.

Sokolowski, R. (1991). The fiduciary relationship and the nature of professions. In E.D. Pellegrino, R.M. Veatch & J.P. Langan (eds) *Ethics, trust, and the professions* (pp. 23–43). Washington: Georgetown University Press.

10 Environmental and social contexts

Richard Fleming

Learning outcomes

1 Outline principles of sound environmental design that enable maximising abilities and support limitations.

2 Describe the application of evidence-based designs in varying contexts: the home, community, residential care and acute care.

3 Discuss the application of principles of participatory involvement to the design of buildings for people with dementia.

4 Discuss how an interprofessional education and interprofessional practice approach may enhance environmental design and participatory engagement.

Key terms

- environmental design

- interprofessional education (IPE)

- interprofessional practice (IPP)

- knowledge translation (KT)

Introduction

What do the people who provide care to people with dementia share? Values, attitudes, skills – perhaps; but there is one that they cannot avoid sharing – the building that the person with dementia is occupying.

Environmental design

It seems fair for me to say, after 30 years of working in the field, that the appreciation of the impact of the building on the success of care is somewhat

Environmental design

Environmental design is the process of addressing surrounding environmental factors when devising plans, programs, policies, buildings or products.

limited. This is not because we lack information on how to reduce the disabilities experienced by people with dementia by designing enabling buildings.

In fact, we have the benefit of a reasonably extensive literature on the subject (Fleming & Purandare, 2010; The King's Fund, 2012; Garre-Olmo et al., 2012; Zuidema et al., 2010; van Hoof et al., 2010; Verbeek et al., 2009; Calkins, 2009). The findings from this literature can be organised around 10 principles of **environmental design** (Fleming & Bennett, 2013) and these have been summarised in Table 10.1.

TABLE 10.1 *Principles of environmental design for people with dementia*

PRINCIPLE 1: UNOBTRUSIVELY REDUCE RISKS

People with dementia require an internal and external environment that is safe, secure and easy to move around if they are to make the best of their remaining abilities. However, obvious safety features and barriers will lead to frustration, agitation and anger, and so potential risks need to be reduced unobtrusively.

PRINCIPLE 2: PROVIDE A HUMAN SCALE

The scale of a building will have an effect on the behaviour and feelings of a person with dementia. The experience of scale is determined by three factors: the number of people that the person encounters, the overall size of the building and the size of the individual components, such as doors, rooms and corridors. A person should not be intimidated by the size of the surroundings or confronted with a multitude of interactions and choices. Rather the scale should help the person feel in control.

PRINCIPLE 3: ALLOW PEOPLE TO SEE AND BE SEEN, AND PROVIDE VISUAL ACCESS TO FREQUENTLY USED LOCATIONS

An environment that allows people to see their destination will help to minimise confusion. It should also enable staff to see patients from where they spend most of their time. This assists with the monitoring of the patients and reassures patients of their safety.

PRINCIPLE 4: REDUCE UNHELPFUL STIMULATION

Because dementia reduces the ability to focus on only those things that are important, a person with dementia can become stressed by prolonged exposure to large amounts of stimulation. The environment should be designed to minimise exposure to stimuli that are not helpful. The full range of senses must be considered. Too much visual stimulation, for example, is as stressful as too much auditory stimulation.

PRINCIPLE 5: OPTIMISE HELPFUL STIMULATION

Ensuring that items that the patient needs to be aware of are strongly highlighted will increase the chance of them being noticed and used. Providing multiple cues using vision, hearing, smell and touch will help to compensate for sensory losses.

PRINCIPLE 6: SUPPORT MOVEMENT AND ENGAGEMENT, INSIDE AND OUTSIDE

Aimless wandering can be minimised by providing a well-defined pathway, free of obstacles and complex decision points, to guide people past points of interest. It also gives them opportunities to engage in activities or social interaction. The pathway should be both internal and external, providing an opportunity and reason to go outside when the weather permits.

》

PRINCIPLE 7: CREATE A FAMILIAR SPACE

The person with dementia is more able to use and enjoy spaces and objects that were familiar to them in their early life. The environment should afford them the opportunity to maintain their competence through the use of familiar furniture, fittings and colours. The involvement of the person with dementia in personalising the environment with their own familiar objects should be encouraged.

PRINCIPLE 8: PROVIDE A VARIETY OF SPACES TO BE ALONE OR WITH OTHERS

People with dementia need to be able to choose to be on their own or spend time with others. This requires the provision of a variety of spaces that prompt a range of activities, e.g. reading alone, conversing with one or two others or engaging in larger group activities.

PRINCIPLE 9: PROVIDE LINKS TO THE COMMUNITY

Without constant reminders of who they were and are, a person with dementia will lose their sense of identity. The best people to remind them are their family and friends. The environment should therefore provide comfortable opportunities for visitors to spend time interacting with the patient.

PRINCIPLE 10: SUPPORT THE VALUES AND GOALS OF CARE

An environment that embodies the values and goals of care, e.g. provides opportunities for engagement with the ordinary activities of daily living to support rehabilitation goals, will assist the person with dementia to respond appropriately, and the staff to deliver the desired care.

The relevance of these principles to the quality of life of people with dementia in residential care has been evaluated in a study involving 275 residents in 35 aged care homes (Fleming et al., 2014). The quality of the environment in these homes was assessed by the use of an audit tool (Fleming, 2011; Fleming, Forbes & Bennett, 2003) based on the 10 principles outlined in Table 10.1 and the quality of life of the residents was assessed by the use of the Dementia Quality of Life (DEMQOL) assessment tool (Smith et al., 2007). Analyses utilising linear regression controlling for a wide range of variables (including gender, age, severity of dementia, medication usage, physical incapacities, number of psychiatric diagnoses and a measure of ability to engage in activities of daily living), identified a significant association between the scores of the global quality of life item of the DEMQOL and the scores of Fleming's Environmental Audit Tool. The quality of the environment, as measured by the Environmental Audit Tool total score, accounted for 14.6% of the variance in quality of life. Further analysis revealed that the provision for alternatives to wandering, familiarity, provision of spaces for privacy and social interaction, and provision of opportunities for engagement in domestic activities were the significant environmental characteristics that contributed to self-reported quality of life.

The quality of the environment was in fact the second best predictor of quality of life, only beaten by the ability of the person with dementia to be involved in activities of daily living – an ability that cannot be expressed without the availability of an environment to support them. While this is relatively new research, the evidence for the positive influence of the environment on a wide range of individual problems, such as disorientation and agitation, has been around for a long time. So why is it that so many people with dementia live in unsatisfactory aged care homes? One way of unravelling the problem is to look at it from a knowledge translation point of view.

Applying knowledge translation

Knowledge translation (KT) is the process of putting knowledge into practice (Straus, Tetroe & Graham, 2009). There are many views and theories on how

> **Knowledge translation (KT)**
> Knowledge translation is the term often used to describe integration of research into practice where the intent is clear from the beginning of the research (Johnson, 2005).

this might be achieved; in fact it has been estimated that there are more than 90 terms used to describe this process (Straus, Tetroe & Graham, 2009). One of the most straightforward and useful models describes the process as occurring in four stages. If knowledge is to be translated into practice, the potential knowledge users must first become aware of is the existence of the evidence for example, by reading an article or attending a class. In the second stage, the users must evaluate the new knowledge and come to the conclusion that it is credible, and that they agree with it. In the third stage, the knowledge must be adopted into practice and in the fourth stage – adherence – the new application becomes business as usual, often as the result of the development of regulations to ensure compliance with accepted good practice (Pathman et al., 1996).

This model of KT was used in an investigation of the obstacles to the application of our knowledge on designing aged care homes for people with dementia (Fleming, Fay & Robinson, 2012). Ten Australian aged care homes, which had recently completed renovations to make them more suitable for people with dementia, were identified, and their managers and architects agreed to participate in the study. The quality of the environment was assessed by the use of an audit tool based on the 10 principles outlined in Table 10.1 (Fleming, 2011; Fleming, Forbes & Bennett, 2003). The managers and architects responsible for the renovations were interviewed to establish their awareness of, and agreement with, the principles. Five of the managers were quite well aware of the principles and agreed with them. All of the architects claimed to be familiar with the principles and agreed with them. Analysis of the difference in the audit tool scores revealed that those facilities that had been renovated by teams comprising an architect and manager, who were aware of and agreed with the principles, scored significantly better than those renovated by teams in which the manager was not aware of the principles. This positive result was quite surprising as it is difficult to get a statistically significant difference in such a small sample.

The result could not be explained in terms of problems with the construction process, cost or corporate policies, as the responses to the structured interviews showed no difference in the impact of these variables on the renovations.

This small study sheds some light on the importance of awareness of new knowledge. The renovations that took place under the control of managers who were not aware of the principles were significantly poorer than those controlled by managers who knew about the principles. This is perhaps not a surprising finding. However, all of the teams had at least one stakeholder – the architect – who did know about the principles. So the team as a whole could be said to have been aware of the knowledge but the influence of the key stakeholder – the manager – appears to have overridden a move to good practice.

On one hand, this suggests that the solution to the problem is to ensure that all managers of aged care homes, who are very often nurses, are educated in how to use the built environment as a tool for improving the quality of life of people with dementia. On the other hand, it can be argued that this knowledge was available and the problem lies in the lack of collaboration between the professions, nurses and architects. This would seem to be a situation which could be improved by a willingness to adopt interprofessional learning (IPL), summarised by the Australasian Interprofessional Practice and Educational Network (n.d.) as:

> a philosophical stance, embracing lifelong learning, adult learning principles and an ongoing, active learning process, between different cultures and health care disciplines. IPL philosophy supports health professionals working collaboratively in a health care setting, through a purposeful interaction with service users and carers, to produce quality patient centred care. It acknowledges both formal and informal methods of learning which progress to develop service delivery.

The wider environment

The positive effects of a well-designed environment extend beyond the aged care home into a person's own home and even into the garden. There are excellent resources available to illustrate this and to provide specific advice on how to create environments that are both prosthetic, that is, they support lost function, and salutogenic, that is, they promote health and well-being (Dementia Services Development Centre, n.d.).

While there is much less research available on the impact of hospital environments on people with dementia, new research is going on in this area (Mazzei, Gillan & Cloutier, 2014) and generalisations are being made from the residential aged care findings to provide advice on how to make the best of the alienating world of acute care (Waller, 2012).

The new frontier is the design of the dementia friendly community (DFC). The recognition of the enormous issue of the doubling of the number of people with dementia over the next 25 years (Australian Institute of Health and Welfare, 2012), the economic implications of providing services and the preference that most people have for being cared for at home has resulted in a widespread enthusiasm for developing DFCs. This idea has been energetically pursued in Japan since 2008 (Takeda, Tanaka & Chiba, 2010), and picked up in the UK's Alzheimer's Society's *Delivering on Dementia: Our Strategy 2012–17* (Alzheimer's Society, 2012), which is being given strong support by the UK government (Older People and Dementia Team, 2012). In 2014, the establishment of DFCs became the top priority for Alzheimer's Australia (Alzheimer's Australia, 2014a).

Involving the dementia community

In 2003, pioneering work on understanding the contribution of the built environment to making communities dementia friendly was published in the UK and has continued to be developed (Mitchell & Burton, 2010; Mitchell et al., 2003). It has provided a foundation for the provision of a number of checklists that can be used to identify the presence or absence of characteristics that are thought to be helpful to people with dementia trying to go about their everyday life (Alzheimer's Australia, 2014b).

This work is remarkable, not only because it foreshadowed interest in developing DFCs, but also because it involved people with dementia in the research. The researchers walked around cities and towns with people with dementia and encouraged them to identify those parts of the environment that were either helpful or unhelpful.

Sadly, the general recognition that people with a disability have a right to participate in decisions about their lives is quite new. Charlton begins his 1998 paradigm shifting book, *Nothing About Us Without Us* with these words (p. ix):

> The lived oppression that people with disabilities have experienced and
> continue to experience is a human rights tragedy of epic proportions. Only in
> the last few decades has this begun to be recognised and resisted. Today, in

fact, we are witnessing a profound sea change among people with disabilities. For the first time, a movement of people with disabilities has emerged in every region of the world which is demanding a recognition of their human rights and their central role in determining those rights.

In a presentation to a conference on consumer directed care in 2013, the chief executive of Alzheimer's Australia noted that it was only in 2000 when his organisation began to involve people with dementia in the life of the organisation (Rees, 2013). At about the same time, researchers in the US were recognising that the very nature of the instruments they used excluded people with a disability from active participation in research (Meyers & Andresen, 2000).

The interprofessional education and interprofessional practice approach

So the involvement of people with dementia in walking around towns and cities with researchers and explaining to them, as partners in the research, the impact of what they saw, felt and heard, was ground breaking. While being an example of participatory action research rather than **interprofessional education (IPE)**, this approach certainly embodied the spirit behind the definition of IPE offered by the Centre for the Advancement of Interprofessional Education (CAIPE).

Barr (1997) states that CAIPE uses the term 'interprofessional education' to include all such learning in academic and work-based settings before and after qualification, adopting an inclusive view of 'professional'.

So what has all of this to do with improving the quality of life of people with dementia by improving the design of the buildings they live in and use? It seems to me that the central values of IPE, as expressed by CAIPE (2014) and summarised below, provide a framework for understanding what needs to be done.

> **Interprofessional education (IPE)**
> Interprofessional education occurs when two or more professions learn with, from and about each other to improve collaboration and the quality of care (http://www.caipe.org.uk/about-us/defining-ipe/).
>
> When students from two or more professions learn about, from and with each other to enable effective collaboration and improve health outcomes (WHO, 2010).

IPE values:

- focus on the needs of individuals, families and communities to improve their quality of care, health outcomes and well-being (keeping best practice central throughout all teaching and learning);
- apply equal opportunities within and between the professions and all with whom they learn and work (acknowledging but setting aside differences in power and status between professions);

- respect individuality, difference and diversity within and between the professions, and all with whom they learn and work (utilising distinctive contributions to learning and practice);
- sustain the identity and expertise of each profession (presenting each profession positively and distinctively);
- promote parity between professions in the learning environment (agreeing 'ground rules');
- instil interprofessional values and perspectives throughout uniprofessional and multiprofessional learning (permeating means and ends for the professional learning in which it is embedded).

We need to recognise that everyone who works, lives in, is treated in or uses the building has a stake in making sure that it is designed to improve quality of care, health outcomes and well-being. While they may not all be professionals in the sense that they are paid and educated to provide a particular service, they should have an equal opportunity to provide input, without reference to the current power and status differences. Their individuality, difference and diversity should be recognised as potential contributions to learning about their needs and how the building will help them to be met. Their individual identity and expertise must be recognised and supported by the development of systems and processes (ground rules) that will result in their views being taken into account in the design.

The example of the improvement in the quality of the design that occurred when the architects and the managers shared their views on the application of the available evidence provides some indication of the results that can be expected when two professions share their expertise in a collaborative effort. It opens up the question of how much better buildings will be when we have afforded people with dementia the same status as a professional and included them in the IPE (the learning with, from and about each other) that is central to research and the creative design process.

However, we must not expect this to be an easy task. There is little research available on the systems, processes and outcomes associated with engagement and participation of users in this type of task. The results of one of the largest and lengthiest studies involving people with disabilities and their families in the development of services provides a cautionary tale (Ottmann, Laragy & Damonze, 2009). The study took place in the Australian capital, Canberra, over a four-year period. While described as a participatory action research study, the values underpinning it, and the activities it involved, seem to be congruent with the IPL values described above. The goal was to evaluate the impact of a participatory action research (PAR)-inspired methodology used to develop a consumer-directed community care/individualised funding service model for people with disabilities – a model of funding that is now being applied in community services for people with dementia. The project produced mixed results, and some of the difficulties were attributed to the gap between the vision and the actuality.

Whereas PAR-inspired methodologies are ideally suited to bringing together key stakeholder groups in negotiation, participation is far from a given. Indeed, PAR is rooted in a vision of a romanticised ideal community, in which people come together in the pursuit of the common good, get along, work collectively towards a collectively agreed upon goal and transform society in the process. However, more often than not, the reality is rather different. Incompatible personalities, differing opinions and world views, as well as competing interests, undermine collective endeavours. Participants who are willing to contribute to the research venture compete with other, more pressing priorities. In other words, to foster and sustain participation over extended periods of time can be hard work (Ottmann et al., 2009, p 40).

Conclusion

It seems likely that the application of IPE principles, perhaps especially in the real–world context of a work-based setting discussed here, will also be hard work.

Self-directed learning activities

Interprofessional practice (IPP)
Occurs when all members of the health service delivery team participate in the team's activities and rely on one another to accomplish common goals and improve health care delivery, thus improving the patient's quality experience (Australasian Interprofessional Practice and Education Network, 2011).

Case study

You are the manager of an aged care facility that is about to be renovated to provide a high quality environment for people with dementia. One of the wings will become a dementia-specific unit. You see this as an opportunity to apply the principles of **interprofessional practice** so that you not only build a good building but build a good team – a team who understands the role that a well-designed building can play in the care of people with dementia and will be able to utilise it to the full when it is built.

Reflective questions

1   Where will you go to gather the evidence that you need to guide the design process?
2   What are the care outcomes that you are aiming for?
3   Who will you invite to join the interprofessional team?
4   How will you instil in them the interprofessional values that you want to drive the team?
5   How will you sustain the identity and expertise of the individuals that make up the team?
6   What systems and processes will you put in place to support the team and to ensure that the views expressed will be taken into account in the design process?
7   How will you deal with, or preferably avoid, the pitfalls of working with such a diverse team? (Hint: the article describing the participant action research study contains some practical advice on how to do this.)
8   How will you know when you have succeeded?
9   How will you celebrate your successes and learn from your failures?

References

Alzheimer's Australia. (2014a). *Dementia enabling environments.* Retrieved 14 October 2014 from http://www.enablingenvironments.com.au/

Alzheimer's Australia. (2014b). *Creating dementia-friendly communities checklists.* Retrieved 15 October 2014 from https://fightdementia.org.au/sites/default/files/checklist_1.pdf

Alzheimer's Society. (2012). *Delivering on dementia: Our strategy 2012–17.* London: Alzheimer's Society.

Australasian Interprofessional Practice and Education Network.(n.d.). *What is IPE/IPL/IPP?* Retrieved 15 October 2014 from http://www.aippen.net/what-is-ipe-ipl-ipp

Australian Institute of Health and Welfare. (2012). *Dementia in Australia: National data analysis and development.* Canberra: AIHW.

Barr, H. (1997). *Interprofessional education – A definition.* CAIPE Bulletin No. 13. Fareham: CAIPE.

Calkins, M.P. (2009). Evidence-based long term care design. *NeuroRehabilitation,* 25(3): 145–54.

Centre for the Advancement of Interprofessional Education (CAIPE). (2014). *Principles of Interprofessional Education.* Retrieved 15 October 2014 from http://caipe.org.uk/resources/principles-of-interprofessional-education/

Charlton, J.I. (1998). *Nothing about us without us: Disability oppression and empowerment.* Berkeley and Los Angeles, CA: University of California Press.

Dementia Services Development Centre. (n.d.). *DSDC: The Dementia Centre.* Retrieved 14 October 2014 from http://www.dementia.stir.ac.uk/

Fleming, R. (2011). An environmental audit tool suitable for use in homelike facilities for people with dementia. *Australasian Journal on Ageing,* 30(3): 108–12.

Fleming, R. & Bennett, K. (2013). Environments that enhance dementia care: Issues and challenges. In R. Nay, S. Garratt, & D. Fetherstonhaugh (eds) *Older People: Issues and innovations in care.* (pp. 411–32) Chatswood, NSW: Elsevier Australia.

Fleming, R., Fay, R. & Robinson, A. (2012). Evidence-based facilities design in health care: A study of aged care facilities in Australia. *Health Services Management Research,* 25: 121–8.

Fleming, R., Forbes, I. & Bennett, K. (2003). *Adapting the ward for people with dementia.* Sydney: NSW Department of Health.

Fleming, R., Goodenough, B., Low, L-F., Chenoweth, L. & Brodaty, H. (2014). The relationship between the quality of the built environment and the quality of life of people with dementia in residential care. *Dementia.* Published online before print. Retrieved 5 May 2014. doi: 10.1177/1471301214532460

Fleming, R. & Purandare, N. (2010). Long-term care for people with dementia: Environmental design guidelines. *International Psychogeriatrics,* 22(7): 1084–96.

Garre-Olmo, J., López-Pousa, S., Turon-Estrada, A., Juvinyà, D., Ballester, D. & Vilalta-Franch, J. (2012). Environmental determinants of quality of life in nursing home residents with severe dementia. *Journal of the American Geriatrics Society,* 60(7): 1230–6.

Mazzei, F., Gillan, R. & Cloutier, D. (2014). Exploring the influence of environment on the spatial behavior of older adults in a purpose-built acute care dementia unit. *American Journal of Alzheimer's Disease and Other Dementias,* June, 29(4): 311–19.

Meyers, A.R. & Andresen, E.M. (2000). Enabling our instruments: Accommodation, universal design, and access to participation in research. *Archives of Physical Medicine and Rehabilitation,* 81 (Supplement 2): S5–S9.

Mitchell, L. & Burton, E. (2010). Designing dementia-friendly neighbourhoods: Helping people with dementia to get out and about. *Journal of Integrated Care,* 18(6): 11–18.

Mitchell, L., Burton, E., Raman, S., Blackman, T., Jenks, M., & Williams, K. (2003). Making the outside world dementia-friendly: Design issues and considerations. *Environment and Planning B: Planning and Design,* 30(4): 605–32.

Older People and Dementia Team. (2012). *Prime Minister's challenge on dementia – delivering major improvements in dementia care and research by 2015.* Leeds: Department of Health.

Ottmann, G., Laragy, C. & Damonze, G. (2009). Consumer participation in designing community based consumer-directed disability care: Lessons from a participatory action research-inspired project. *Systemic Practice and Action Research,* 22(1): 31–44.

Pathman, D.E., Konrad, T.R., Freed, G.L., Freeman, V.A. & Koch, G.G. (1996). The awareness-to-adherence model of the steps to clinical guideline compliance: The case of pediatric vaccine recommendations. *Medical Care*, 34(9): 873–89.

Rees, G. (2013). 'Consumer directed care and dementia', paper presented at the Delivering Consumer Directed Aged Care Conference Crown Promenade, Melbourne, 21 May 2013.

Smith, S.C., Lamping, D.L., Banerjee, S., Harwood, R.H., Foley, B., Smith, P. .... Knapps, M. (2007). Development of a new measure of health-related quality of life for people with dementia: DEMQOL. *Psychological Medicine*, 37(05): 737–46.

Straus, S.E., Tetroe, J. & Graham, I. (2009). Defining knowledge translation. *Canadian Medical Association Journal*, 181(3–4): 165–8.

Takeda, A., Tanaka, N. & Chiba, T. (2010). Prospects of future measures for persons with dementia in Japan. *Psychogeriatrics*, 10(2): 95–101.

The King's Fund. (2012). *Developing supportive design for people with dementia: Overarching design principles*. London: The King's Fund.

van Hoof, J., Kort, H.S., van Waarde, H. & Blom, M.M. (2010). Environmental interventions and the design of homes for older adults with dementia: An overview. *American Journal of Alzheimer's Disease and Other Dementias*, 25(3): 202–32.

Verbeek, H., van Rossum, E., Zwakhalen, S.M., Kempen, G.I. & Hamers, J.P. (2009). Small, homelike care environments for older people with dementia: A literature review. *International Psychogeriatrics*, 21(2): 252–64.

Waller, S. (2012). Redesigning wards to support people with dementia in hospital. *Nursing Older People*, 24(2): 16–21.

Zuidema, S.U., de Jonghe, J.F., Verhey, F.R. & Koopmans, R.T. (2010). Environmental correlates of neuropsychiatric symptoms in nursing home patients with dementia. *International Journal of Geriatric Psychiatry*, 25(1): 14–22.

Conclusion

Dimity Pond

Learning outcomes

1. Discuss ways in which the interprofessional approach might assist individuals with dementia and carers at each stage of the dementia journey.

2. Discuss ways in which individuals with dementia and their carers can contribute to the work of the team at each stage of the journey.

3. Consider how a big team, consisting of a range of professionals with various roles, might work together, particularly in the middle stages where the person living with dementia is requiring maximum support in the home.

4. Discuss the issues relating to leadership in team care and how the team might resolve these issues in different clinical settings.

Key terms

- dementia
- evidence-based practice (EBP)
- leadership

Introduction

Many of the key messages from this book are about how health professionals should work together in the care of people living with **dementia**. To summarise some of the key points, we will follow Mary as she travels along a dementia journey, and explore some of the many ways in which professionals can work together to help her on that journey.

> **Dementia**
> Dementia is now referred to as a neurocognitive disorder (NCD) (American Psychiatric Association, 2013), that is, the result of chronic or progressive damage to the brain.

Early signs of dementia

Mary, aged 76, lives alone. Her husband died shortly after he retired some 10 years ago and the couple had no children. Mary used to work in an office, but has lost touch with most of her former workmates now. Her one companion is a much loved dog named Freddie, although there is also a niece who visits from time to time. She has been a patient of her GP for over 10 years. She books a regular monthly appointment for a blood pressure check, repeats of her eight medications when necessary and a bit of a chat. She has quite stable diabetes, for which she is taking oral medication, and every three months she has this reviewed under a chronic disease management plan. She has never brought along her niece to these appointments.

The GP asks Mary to book a routine annual 75+ Health Assessment to be conducted by the practice nurse. During this assessment, the practice nurse asks Mary if she ever has any problems with her memory. When Mary responds in the affirmative, the nurse administers the Standardized Mini-Mental State Examination (MMSE), which is a brief test of cognitive function (Molloy & Stamdish, 1997). It is scored out of 30 and the cut off is usually 23/24 (i.e. if the person scores 23 or below they are thought to be in need of further assessment for dementia). Mary scores 24. Despite this being in the normal range, the nurse is a bit concerned as she scored 28 in the previous year. The nurse knows Mary quite well, from assisting with her diabetes checks, and feels that Mary is 'not herself', because she seems a bit anxious and more disorganised than usual. She asks Mary for permission to talk to her GP about the interview as well as giving him the health assessment.

Reflective questions

1 What ethical issues arise when the nurse communicates with the GP in this way? Are they resolved by her asking permission to chat to the GP?
2 Are there any other issues that the nurse might cover in Mary's case? What factors influence how far the nurse will go in her own assessment of Mary?

To assist you, see Chapter 1, especially ethical principles, collaborative practice, communication; Chapter 2 on diagnosis of dementia; and Chapter 9 on ethics, especially Figure 9.1, p. 152, on Ethics First Aid © checklist.

Case study ctd.

When Mary goes back to see the GP, he questions her about her memory and also how well she is performing in her usual activities of daily living. She agrees that her memory is not what it was but states that she is managing well at home. 'I don't want to go into a home,' she says tearfully. 'What would I do with Freddie?'

At this point, the GP wonders if Mary might be affected by depression. He asks her the questions on the Geriatric Depression Scale (GDS) (Yesavage et al., 1983) and finds that she scores in the depression range on this. Depression might well account for her poor cognition. She readily agrees that she might be depressed and goes along with a plan to see a psychologist who visits the practice each week. However, she doesn't think it will do much good. 'I'm lonely,' she says. 'I don't know what I would do without Freddie.'

See Chapter 2 on making the diagnosis of dementia.

Reflective questions

1 What other avenues might the GP pursue in the management of Mary's depression and loneliness?
2 Should any other health or community professionals be involved?

To assist you, see Chapters 1 and 8 on person- and relationship-centred care, and Chapter 3 on collaborative practice.

Case study ctd.

Several weeks later, the GP receives a report from the psychologist, whose own testing has found Mary to be both depressed and anxious. She states that Mary is responding well to some simple breathing exercises and positive events scheduling suggested as treatment, and still has a number of treatment sessions to go.

The GP decides to conduct a case conference about Mary with the psychologist and the practice nurse. The case conference is run in the surgery, with the psychologist on the phone and both the GP and the practice nurse attending. Each professional contributes their thoughts about Mary and it is decided that the practice nurse should explore socialisation options with her, to reduce her loneliness. This can easily be done with funding through the practice nurse Medicare item numbers associated with Mary's chronic disease management plan.

When the nurse meets Mary, they run through a number of options, and in the end Mary agrees to join the knitting group that meets weekly in the library, and also visit the community health centre lunch program once a month. The nurse organises attendance to the lunch program over the phone, and gives Mary details about the knitting group. (Note: the 'local context' in Figure 3.3. Different geographical locations will have different activities available.)

At the case conference, the practice nurse had expressed some concerns about Mary managing her medications. As a result, the GP also organises a pharmacy home medications review. This review explores whether Mary understands and manages her medications correctly, looks at the options for reducing the number of medications with available combination tablets and explores whether any of them might be contributing to Mary's forgetfulness. The number of medications is reduced from eight to six daily as a result, and Mary is issued with a Webster-pak, in which the medications are packed in easily accessible doses for each day.

Reflective questions

1 How should the group interact in such a multidisciplinary case conference?
2 Should a leader be explicitly chosen? If so, would it be preferable to assume that the GP is the leader of this group?
3 If you were teaching a student to observe this interaction, what parts of the interactions should the student focus on? How would the student tell if this was a working collaborative group or not?
4 How would you measure the results of this case conference? What factors would you consider? How could these measurements affect future case conferences?

Leadership
Leadership is a process of social influences that maximise the efforts of others towards the achievement of a goal.

To assist you, see the Chapter 3 section on collaborative practice, Chapter 4 on evidence-based practice and Chapter 5 on **leadership**.

Ctd.

Three months' later, the GP asks the nurse to review Mary and complete another MMSE and GDS. Both have improved and are now well within the normal range. Nevertheless, the GP decides to keep a close watch on Mary. He knows that depression in the elderly is often a precursor to dementia.

Middle stage of the dementia journey

The following year, the practice nurse again runs through the 75+ Health Assessment with Mary. As in the previous year, Mary complains that her memory is 'not what it used to be', so the nurse again administers the MMSE. This time Mary scores 21 out of 30. The nurse also runs through the GDS and Mary scores within the normal range. The nurse asks Mary a series of questions about her ability to perform activities of daily living. Mary states that she is coping well but the nurse senses again that things are not as they should be. Mary appears a bit dishevelled and was late for her appointment. She has also lost 5kg in weight compared with her assessment last year. The nurse thinks that it would be ideal if she could talk to another family member who knows Mary well, to find out what is really going on. She suggests this to the GP.

This time, when Mary goes to the GP for her health assessment review she brings her niece, Alison, with her, as requested. The GP explains that the practice is concerned because some of the memory tests are not as good as they were and also because Mary has lost weight. He asks Alison what she thinks about the situation.

Reflective questions

1 Do you think that the GP should have included the practice nurse in this visit with Alison? Why or why not?
2 What would the practice nurse have been able to contribute?
3 What information would have been helpful to the practice nurse in the ongoing management of Mary?

To assist you, see Chapter 3 on collaboration.

Alison responds that she doesn't see Mary every day but she has also noticed that she seems to have lost weight. She says that there is not a lot of food in the refrigerator. She proposes to take Mary up to the local club regularly on Sundays, for the Sunday roast meal that is offered then.

Alison also says Mary rings her up a bit more than usual. Alison's husband, Bob, has taken over Mary's finances, as Mary had got into a bit of a muddle with unpaid bills. Mary had set up Bob and Alison jointly as her legal powers of attorney to make this possible.

The GP asks if other legal documents have all been organised, such as a will and a legal authority for Alison and Bob to make decisions about Mary's health if she became ill. Mary does have a will but both Alison and Mary were interested in pursuing the legal authority (titled differently in different areas), which they had not previously been aware of. They agree to visit Mary's solicitor about this.

The GP also suggests that Mary's symptoms might unfortunately be the first signs of Alzheimer's disease. He asks Mary and Alison if they understand what this is and spends some time explaining it to them. He suggests that Mary sees the geriatrician to explore this further. In the meantime, he says that he needs to do some blood tests and also a computerised tomography (CT) scan to make sure that there are no other physical problems that might be affecting Mary's functioning.

Reflective questions

1 Do you think that the GP should have raised the possibility of Alzheimer's disease at this stage before it is fully diagnosed? Why or why not? (Read Iliffe et al. (2009) for more information about this issue.)
2 Should he have used the words 'Alzheimer's disease' or would 'dementia' have been a better option?
3 How do you think Mary and Alison might be responding to this news emotionally? What other diseases that mimic dementia might the GP be looking for with the blood tests and CT scan? Are these blood tests and CT scan the correct next step according to guidelines? (Read the National Collaborating Centre for Mental Health's NICE–SCIE Guidelines for more information.)
4 What implications would such a diagnosis have for Mary's future?

Evidence-based practice (EBP) Health care professionals who perform evidence-based practice use research evidence along with clinical expertise and patient preferences.

To assist you, see Chapter 9 on ethics and Chapter 4 on **evidence-based practice** (Eccles, North of England evidence-based guidelines development project referenced in Chapter 4).

Ctd.

The GP also says that, at this stage, there is another referral he would like to make, along with the one to the geriatrician. This is to a dietician to review Mary's diet. He suggests that Alison accompanies Mary on this visit, to help Mary remember the advice that she is given.

Four months later

Case study ctd.

Mary and Alison again visit the GP together, and this time the practice nurse attends the visit. The GP runs through the information that he has gathered. The geriatrician assessed Mary and has made a diagnosis of mild dementia. She wrote back to the GP stating that she has started Mary on an anti-dementia medication and suggested that she return for a review in six months' time. Mary found the medication made her feel a bit unwell to start with but she has become used to it now. She is not sure, but thinks that it may be doing her memory some good. The dietician also reviewed Mary and found that her diet was inadequate. In her letter to the GP, she suggested that Mary access Meals on Wheels but Mary is reluctant to do this as she feels that she is managing better now. She has gained 2kg since starting to eat regular weekly meals with Alison. Alison also provides a few frozen home cooked meals for her to eat during the week, using the menus provided by the dietician, and is happy to continue doing this.

The practice nurse raises the issue that Mary might benefit from some home care services. She suggests a home care visitor once a week could do some house cleaning and also assist Mary with the shopping. This would give Alison a break, as she has teenage children to look after, as well as the responsibilities that she has taken on with Mary. Mary rather reluctantly agrees to this but says that she will be very busy tidying up the house before the home care people come.

Reflective questions

1 At what stage is Mary in terms of accepting the Meals on Wheels as a behaviour change? How would you imagine the team might help her move to a different stage?
2 Do you think Mary has full insight into the burden she is placing on Alison? Why or why not? How can the team assist Alison to relieve the carer burden?
3 There are now a large number of people on the team looking after Mary. Make a list of who is involved. Is it likely that there are others not mentioned in the text?
4 Do these people all need to communicate with each other or is it sufficient that they communicate with the GP? How would it be best to organise communication for those who need it?

To assist you, see Chapter 2 on giving out information; Chapter 4, the Procheska and Velicer article on behaviour change and description of it in the chapter (p. 70) and Chapter 6.

Case study ctd.

At this point, the GP suggests that the practice nurse reviews Mary's diabetes care plan, and add a number of people and issues related to dementia to it. Copies of the care plan can be sent, with Mary's consent, to all of the people who are looking after her, so that they are aware of the other members of the team and what issues are being addressed.

When the practice nurse does this, she realises what a burden is being placed on Alison, and rings her to suggest that she attend Alzheimer's Australia's carer support groups. These groups may be attended by the carer and the person living with dementia, and allows carers to discuss issues and how to access various support services.

Eight months later

Case study ctd.

A year has now gone past, and it is time for the 75+ Health Assessment again. Mary is still taking the anti-dementia drugs, as the geriatrician judged that she was better off with these. She is now getting home care services and has agreed to Meals on Wheels. Alison sees her regularly and still takes her to the club for a meal once a week. She has completed the legal documentation required to give Alison and Bob decision-making power if she becomes ill.

The nurse chooses to do the 75+ Health Assessment in Mary's home, with Alison present. The nurse feels that she can get a better impression of how well Mary is coping if she completes this work in the home setting. During the assessment, Mary admits that she has had some falls in recent months. Completion of a falls checklist reveals that she feels unsteady on her feet and has difficulty seeing obstacles in her path on occasions. She also suffers from some degree of urinary urgency, Mary tends to rush to the toilet and sometimes falls in the process. The GP is reluctant to put her on medication for her urinary urgency, as it appears to cause cognitive problems. She scores 19 out of 30 on the MMSE.

After a quick visit around the house, the nurse suggests that Alison work with Mary to declutter the place a little. She also suggests that some loose rugs be taken up and that white masking tape be run along the edge of the stairs to assist Mary with seeing them.

The practice nurse also discusses with Mary and Alison the need for Mary to develop an advance care plan. This plan has agreed strategies in it for eventualities around any deterioration in Mary's health. For example, if Mary was to suffer a heart attack, would she want to be resuscitated? Are there any circumstances which she could foresee when she would be comfortable with a move to residential aged care? Such a plan can help Alison and Bob understand Mary's wishes when they make health care decisions for Mary in the future.

Reflective questions

1 Do you think that the practice nurse should take the initiative in this situation, in reviewing the house for falls risks and in suggesting the advance care plan?
2 What are the advantages and disadvantages of her doing this?

To assist you, see Chapter 5 on leadership and Chapter 6.

Case study ctd.

At the GP follow-up meeting, the following referrals were made:

- to the ophthalmologist to assess Mary's vision;
- to the urologist to explore alternative options to cope with Mary's urinary problems;
- to the aged care assessment team to assess Mary for a government 'package' of care to support her in the home. This included a referral to the occupational therapist, who forms part of the team, to assess Mary and the home in relation to falls and dementia.

The nurse suggests that Mary attend a local falls prevention class run by a physiotherapist once the other referrals are attended.

The GP also discusses the advance care plan that Mary and her relatives have drawn up and makes sure that it is filed in the notes. He talks to Alison and Mary about the way in which dementia progresses and that, as it is a terminal disease, the plan is very important.

Reflective questions

1 Do all the members of the team have to communicate with each other about Mary's problems? What other models of communication might work? What is the role of the general practice in this issue?
2 How is it best to keep them all 'in the loop' about what is happening with Mary? Was it wise for the GP to mention that dementia is a terminal disease? Might this information best be kept from Mary? Could this disclosure have been handled differently?

To assist you, see Chapter 2 on giving out information, Chapter 6 and Chapter 9. Especially consider whether Mary has full rights as a 'person' at this stage.

Later stages of the dementia journey

One year later

Case study ctd.

Another year has gone past and it is time again for Mary's 75+ Health Assessment. Mary is still living at home but experiencing more difficulties coping with everyday living. The aged care assessment team has seen her again during the year and classified her as eligible for admission to residential aged care when the time is right. This classification also gives her eligibility for more hours of support in the home but there are still days when no one visits her.

When the practice nurse again visits the home, Alison is there to meet her. Alison explains that she is feeling the strain as she has had some difficulties with a sick husband as well as supporting her teenage children. She wonders if there is someone who could check on Mary each day, and the nurse explains that the Red Cross has a volunteer service where someone rings each morning to have a chat. If no one answers the phone, they would then ring Alison or a neighbour to check on Mary. Alison is greatly relieved by this and agrees to organise it.

Mary is visibly frailer now and clearly not walking well. Her MMSE score is 15 out of 30. She appears depressed and her beloved Freddie has died during this last 12 months. The house is spotless but Alison explains that she came over the day before to help Mary prepare for the nurse visit. She says that the home care can only do so much and there is often some additional home support needed.

The nurse, Mary and Alison talk about a possible move to residential aged care. This would relieve Mary of the burden of living alone. In her advance care plan, Mary had stated that she would be ready to move to care if she had become doubly incontinent but this is not the case. However, she feels that everything is getting a bit much. It is agreed that Alison will start to explore what nursing homes have vacancies and put Mary's name down on their waiting lists.

When the GP reviews the 75+ Health Assessment, he chats to Mary and Alison about this possible move, and supports them in making this decision. He suggests that Alison look on the internet to find resources to assist her with assessing the facilities that she is visiting.

Six months later, Mary is admitted to residential aged care. Alison had been particularly impressed with a facility that demonstrated patient-centred care (Chapter 8) when she visited it, and also met many of the principles of environmental design for people with dementia (Table 10.1), so this is where Mary moved.

Terminal phase

Case study ctd.

Two years later, the GP reviews Mary in residential aged care. By this time, she is bed bound and has difficulty communicating. She no longer recognises Alison by name although she is always pleased to see her. She is entering the terminal phase of her dementia journey.

The GP discusses this with Alison, who states that she would not be surprised if Mary died within the next 12 months. The GP states that this is a sign that a palliative approach is appropriate for management of any problems that might arise. The advance care plan had already stated that if Mary is unable to recognise her family she would not want any active treatment, not go to hospital and not have any intravenous medication or fluids. Alison readily agrees that these suggestions would apply from now on, in line with the palliative approach to keep Mary comfortable but not to apply any unnecessarily active treatment to prolong life.

The GP asks for a case conference with the facility staff, with Alison present. They spend a little time discussing the advance care plan and reassuring staff that the family is very happy for Mary to die peacefully in the facility, rather than being transported to hospital. The plan is placed at the front of Mary's notes.

Two months later, Mary has a bad choking fit as she tries to swallow dinner. She has been seen by the speech pathologist and a thickened fluid prescribed because she is not swallowing well. However, the swallowing difficulties have progressed as the dementia has progressed, resulting in choking. Mary recovers from the choking episode but rapidly develops a chest infection as some food has clearly entered her lungs. The GP tries some oral antibiotics and notifies the family. Mary rallies briefly then dies peacefully three days later, with Alison and Bob in attendance.

Self-directed learning activities

Prepare a care plan listing team members and what each did to assist Mary with her dementia and dementia related issues.

1 Should Alison be included on the care plan? What evaluation might you include to measure the success of each professional's contribution to the care plan?

2 How might the team reflect on these evaluations in order to modify the care plan when it is reviewed?

3 How might the team support each other in looking after Mary?

To assist you, see Chapter 4 and Chapter 6.

References

Iliffe, S., Robinson, L., Brayne, C, Goodman, G, Rait, G., Manthorpe, J & Ashley, P. (2009). Primary care and dementia: 1. diagnosis, screening and disclosure· *International Journal of Geriatric Psychiatry*, September, 24(9): 895–901. doi: 10.1002/gps.2204

Molloy, D.W. & Standish, T. I (1997). A guide to the Standardized Mini-Mental State Examination. *International Psychogeriatrics*, 9 (Supplement 1): 87–94.

National Collaborating Centre for Mental Health. (n.d.). *A NICE–SCIE Guideline on supporting people with dementia and their carers in health and social care*. National Clinical Practice Guideline Number 42. Retrieved 24 February 2015 from http://www.nice.org.uk/guidance/cg42/evidence/cg42-dementia-full-guideline-including-appendices-172

Yesavage, J.A., Brink, T.L., Rose, T.L., Lum, O., Huang, V., Adey, M. & Leirer, V.O. (1983). Development and validation of a geriatric depression screening scale: A preliminary report. *Journal of Psychiatric Research*, 17(1): 37–49.

Glossary

Aged care services The Australian government subsidises many different types of aged care services to help people stay at home. They are there to help people stay as independent as they can through a system that provides fair and equitable access to services for all older people living in Australia.

Alzheimer's disease Alzheimer's disease is the most common form of major neurocognitive disorder. It was first described by Dr Alois Alzheimer in 1907 as he found particular changes on post-mortem brain examination (American Psychiatric Association, 2013).

Autonomy The capacity to make rational, uncoerced and informed decisions about the things that affect one's life.

Capabilities Forman, Jones & Thistlethwaite (2014) define capability as 'has been used in preference to competence in one IPE framework, as it is considered by some educators to reflect more optimally the necessity that learners and professionals respond and adapt to health care and systems changes'.

Collaborative practice (CP) Communication, sharing and problem solving between the physician and nurse as peers; this pattern of practice also implies a shared responsibility and accountability for patient care.

Communication An exchange of information between individuals using speech, visual aids, body language, writing or behaviour.

Competencies Forman, Jones & Thistlethwaite (2014) define competency as the ability to 'identify specific knowledge, skills, attitudes, values and judgements that are dynamic, developmental and evolutionary'.

Culture The main definition of culture used in this book is: 'Culture is all aspects of life, the totality of meanings, ideas and beliefs shared by individuals within a group of people. Culture is learned, it includes language, values, norms, customs. (http://www.design.iastate.edu/NAB/about/thinkingskills/cultural_context/cultural.html).

Dementia Dementia is now referred to as a neurocognitive disorder (NCD) (American Psychiatric Association, 2013), that is, the result of chronic or progressive damage to the brain.

Environmental design Environmental design is the process of addressing surrounding environmental factors when devising plans, programs, policies, buildings or products.

Ethics The body of values and judgements relating to human conduct, especially with respect to the rightness and wrongness of certain actions, and to the motives and ends of such actions.

Evaluation Appraisal or value of something.

Evidence-based practice (EBP) Health care professionals who perform evidence-based practice use research evidence along with clinical expertise and patient preferences.

Integrated approach Leutz (1999) defines the integrated approach to care as: 'The search to connect the healthcare system (acute, primary medical and skilled) with other human service systems (e.g. long-term care, education and vocational and housing services) to improve outcomes (clinical, satisfaction and efficiency)'.

Interprofessional The terms 'interprofessional education/practice/teamwork' etc. have been defined by various groups. These terms are often used interchangeably. Where we simply use the term 'interprofessional', we do so when two or more professions are working collaboratively together.

Interprofessional collaboration (IPC) Cited in* Nisbet et al. The process of developing and maintaining effective interprofessional working relationships with learners, practitioners, patients/clients/families and communities to enable optimal health outcomes (Canadian Interprofessional Health Collaborative, 2010, p. 8).

Interprofessional education (IPE) Interprofessional education occurs when two or more professions learn with, from and about each other to improve collaboration and the quality of care (http://www.caipe.org.uk/about-us/defining-ipe/).

Interprofessional education (IPE) Cited in ** IECEP When students from two or more professions learn about, from and with each other to enable effective collaboration and improve health outcomes (WHO, 2010).

Interprofessional practice (IPP) Cited in* Nisbet et al. Occurs when all members of the health service delivery team participate in the team's activities and rely on one

another to accomplish common goals and improve health care delivery, thus improving the patient's quality experience (Australasian Interprofessional Practice and Education Network, 2011).

Interprofessional teamwork Cited in IECEP** The levels of cooperation, coordination and collaboration characterising the relationships between professions in delivering patient-centred care.

Knowledge translation (KT) Knowledge translation is the term often used to describe integration of research into practice where the intent is clear from the beginning of the research (Johnson, 2005).

Leadership Leadership is a process of social influences that maximise the efforts of others towards the achievement of a goal.

Neurocognitive disorder (NCD) Neurocognitive disorder is an umbrella term to describe a collection of disease processes that cause different sequences of brain damage, and variations in appearance and severity of symptoms (American Psychiatric Association, 2013).

Palliative care Palliative care is an approach that improves the quality of life of patients and their families facing the problems associated with life-threatening illness, through the prevention and relief of suffering by means of early identification and impeccable assessment and treatment of pain and other problems; physical, psychosocial and spiritual.

Patient-focused care Providing care that is respectful of and responsive to individual patient preferences, needs and values, and ensuring that patient values guide all clinical decisions.

Person-centred care Person-centred care is the 'treatment and care provided by health services which place the person at the centre of their own care and considers the needs of the older person's carers' (Victorian Government Department of Human Services, 2003).

Personality Personality is made up of the characteristic patterns of thoughts, feelings and behaviours that make a person unique. It arises from within the individual and remains fairly consistent throughout life.

Personhood The state or fact of being an individual or having human characteristics and feelings.

Power Power, it has been argued, is the ability or capacity to act or to exercise influence. As such, it has many dimensions (gender, race, class, knowledge, etc.) that can impact on interprofessional relations (Baker et al., 2011).

Relationship-centred care Relationship-centred care is care in which all participants appreciate

the importance of their relationships with one another (Beach, C., Inui, T. & the Relationship-Centred Care Research Network, 2006).

Resilience Individual resilience is the ability to bounce back from negative emotional experiences and flexible adaptation to the changing demands of stressful experiences (Tugade & Fredrickson, 2004).

Respect Due regard for the feelings, wishes or rights of others.

Sustainability Sustainability is the endurance of systems and processes.

Teamwork Teamwork is the process of working collaboratively with a group of people in order to achieve a goal.

Value The regard that something is held to deserve; the importance, worth or usefulness of something.

References

American Psychiatric Association. (2013). *Diagnostic and Statistical Manual of Mental Disorders* (5th edn). Arlington, VA: APA.

Baker, L., Egan-Lee, E., Martimianakis, M.A. & Reeves, S. (2011). Relationships of power: Implications for interprofessional education. *Journal of Interprofessional Care*, March, 25(2): 98–104.

Beach, C., Inui, T. & the Relationship-Centred Care Research Network. (2006). Relationship-centred care. A constructive reframing. *Journal of General Internal Medicine*, 21 (Supplement 1): S3–S8.

Forman, D., Jones, M. & Thistlethwaite, J. (eds). (2014). *Leadership development for interprofessional education and collaborative practice*. Basingstoke: Palgrave Macmillan.

** Interprofessional Education Collaborative Expert Panel (IECEP). (2011). *Core competencies for interprofessional collaborative practice: Report of an expert panel*. Washington, DC: Interprofessional Education Collaborative.

Johnson, L.S. (2005). From knowledge transfer to knowledge translation: Applying research to practice. *OT Now*, July/August, 11–14.

Leutz, W.N. (1999). Five laws for integrating medical and social services: Lessons from the United States and the United Kingdom. *Milbank Quarterly*, 77(1): 77–110.

* Nisbet, G., Lee, A., Kumar, K., Thistlethwaite, J. & Dunston, R. (2011). *Interprofessional Health Education – A literature review: Overview of international and Australian developments in interprofessional health education*. Sydney: Centre for Research in Learning and Change, University of Technology.

Tugade, M.M. & Fredrickson, B.L. (2004). Resilient individuals use positive emotions to bounce back from negative emotional experiences. *Journal of Personality and Social Psychology*, 86: 320–33.

Victorian Government Department of Human Services. (2003). *Improving care for older people: A policy for health services*. Retrieved 7 July 2014 from http://www. health.vic.gov.au

Appendix

Information about dementia and dementia care

There are many books and resources currently available about dementia and dementia care. Below we have listed some that you might find useful but this is by no means exhaustive.

Books

Bannergee, S. & Lawrence, V. (2010). *Managing dementia in a multicultural society.* Chichester: Wiley-Blackwell.

Boss, P. (2011). *Loving someone who has dementia: How to find hope while coping with stress and grief.* San Francisco: Jossey-Bass.

Bromage, A., Clouder, L., Thistlethwaite, J. & Gordon, F. (2010). *Interprofessional e-learning and collaborative work: Practices and technologies.* New York: Information Science Reference.

Clarke, C., Wilkinson, H., Keady, J. & Gibb, C. (2011). *Risk assessment and management for living well with dementia.* London: Jessica Kingsley.

Crawford, K. (2011). *Interprofessional collaboration in social work practice.* London: Sage.

Cox, C. (2007). *Dementia and social work practice research and intervention.* New York: Springer Publishing.

Forman, D., Jones, M. & Thistlethwaite, J. (eds). (2014). *Leadership development for interprofessional education and collaborative practice.* Basingstoke: Palgrave Macmillan.

Gautier, S. & Rosa-Neto, P. (2011). *Case studies in dementia: Common and uncommon presentations.* New York: Cambridge University Press.

Gillard, J. & Marshall, M. (2012). *Transforming the quality of life for people with dementia through contact with the natural world: Fresh air on my face.* London: Jessica Kingsley.

Gitlin, L. & Corcoran, M. (2005). *Occupational therapy and dementia care: The home environmental skill-building program for individuals and families.* Bethesda, MD: American Occupational Therapy Association.

Goodman, B. & Clemow, R. (2010). *Nursing and collaborative practice: A guide to interprofessional learning and working.* London: Learning Matters.

Hughes, J. (2011). *Thinking through dementia.* Oxford: Oxford University Press.

Innes, A. & Hatfield, K. (2002). *Healing arts therapies and person-centred dementia care*. Philadelphia: Jessica Kingsley.

James, I. (2011). *Understanding behaviour in dementia that challenges: A guide to assessment and treatment*. London: Jessica Kingsley.

Jewell, A. (2011). *Spirituality and personhood in dementia*. Philadelphia: Jessica Kingsley.

Koubel, G. & Bungay, H. (2012). *Rights, risks and responsibilities: Interprofessional work in health and social care*. Basingstoke: Palgrave Macmillan.

Littlechild, B. & Smith, B. (2012). *A handbook for interprofessional practice in the human services: Learning to work together*. London: Pearson.

Mace, N.L. & Rabins, P.V. (1981). *The 36-hour day: A family guide to caring for people who have Alzheimer disease, related dementias, and memory loss* (5th edn). Baltimore, MD: Johns Hopkins University Press.

Martin, G. & Sabbagh, M. (2011). *Palliative care for advanced Alzheimer's and dementia: Guidelines and standards for evidence-based care*. New York: Springer Publishing Co.

Mast, B. (2011). *Whole person dementia assessment*. Baltimore, MD: Health Professions Press.

McCarthy, B. (2011). *Hearing the person with dementia: Person-centred approaches to communication for families and caregivers*. London: Jessica Kingsley.

McCurry, S. & Drossel, C. (2011). *Treating dementia in context: A step by step guide to working with individuals and families*. Washington, DC: American Psychological Association.

Oddy, R. (2011). *Promoting the mobility of people with dementia: A problem solving approach* (3rd edn). London: Alzheimer's Association.

Pool, J. (2012). *The Pool Activity Level (PAL) instrument for occupational profiling: A practical resource for carers of people with cognitive impairment* (4th edn). London: Jessica Kingsley.

Quinney, A. & Halford-Letchfield, T. (2012). *Interprofessional social work: Effective collaborative approaches*. London: Learning Matters.

Standing, M. (2010). *Clinical judgement and decision making in nursing and interprofessional healthcare*. Maidenhead: Open University Press.

Thistlethwaite, J. (2012). *Values-based interprofessional collaborative practice: Working together in health care*. Cambridge: Cambridge University Press.

Trod, L. & Chivers, L. (2011). *Interprofessional working in practice: Learning and working together for children and families*. Maidenhead: Open University Press.

Whitworth, H. & Whitworth, J. (2011). *A caregiver's guide to Lewy body dementia*. New York: Demos Health.

Wu, J. (2011). *Early detection and rehabilitation technologies for dementia neuroscience and biomedical applications*. Hershey: Medical information Science.

Associations and resource centres

You are encouraged to look at the lists below to gain a wider appreciation of interprofessional education and practice.

International interprofessional networks

AIHC	American Interprofessional Health Collaborative: www.aihc-us.org/
AIPPEN	Australasian Interprofessional Practice and Education Network: www.aippen.net
ATBH	All Together Better Health: http://www.atbh7.pitt.edu/
CAIPE	Centre for the Advancement of Interprofessional Education: www.caipe.org.uk
CIHC	Canadian Interprofessional Health Collaborative: www.cihc.ca/
EIPEN	European Interprofessional Practice and Education Network: www.eipen.eu/
InterEd	International Association for Interprofessional Education and Collaborative Practice: http://solr.bccampus.ca:8001/bcc/items/f0a17c33-b09f-eecb-3634-a829d3f70686/1/
JAIPE	Japan Association for Interprofessional Education: www.jaipe.net/
NIPNET	Nordic Interprofessional Network: www.nipnet.org/
The Network: TUFH	The Network: Towards Unity for Health: http://www.the-networktufh.org/

Resource centres

Alzheimer's Australia lists a number of useful dementia websites: http://www.fightdementia.org.au/about-dementia-and-memory-loss/resources/useful-websites

Australian Dementia Study Training Centres also have useful resources on their websites, including training materials for health care teams and carers: http://www.dtsc.com.au/

Canadian Coalition for Global Health Research: http://www.ccghr.ca/

Dementia Collaborative Research Centres have many useful resources on their websites, including questionnaires and research reports: http://www.dementiaresearch.org.au/

Dementia Services Development Centre is a UK centre for training and development in dementia care: http://dementia.stir.ac.uk

Higher Education Academy, Health Sciences and Practice Subject Centre works with the wider health professions community to contribute to policy development and implementation: http://www.health.heacademy.ac.uk

Weblinks

The following weblinks provide further information about dementia, interprofessional education and collaborative practice.

14 Essentials is a self-paced teaching aid that gives information and practical tips about each key element: http://www.dementiaresearch.org.au/14-essentials-online-learning.html

Aged Rights Advocacy Service: Residential care: http://www.sa.agedrights.asn.au/residential_care/preventing_elder_abuse/rights_of_older_person

Alzheimer's Association's (US) position on a number of ethical, medical and care topics related to Alzheimer's disease and dementia: http://www.alz.org/about_us_statements.asp

National Human Rights Action Plan: Older people: http://www.humanrightsactionplan.org.au/nhrap/focus-area/older-people

Nuffield Council on Bioethics: Dementia: ethical issues: http://nuffieldbioethics.org/project/dementia/

Office of Learning and Teaching: resources – interprofessional education in health: http://www.olt.gov.au/search

Patient-centered care improvement guide: http://www.patient-centeredcare.org/

United Nations notes on legal capacity and forced interventions: http://www.un.org/esa/socdev/enable/rights/ahc8docs/ahc8idc1218ex.doc

WHO IPE Framework: http://www.who.int/hrh/resources/framework_action/en/

Wicking TACF interprofessional clinical placement curriculum document: http://www.utas.edu.au/wicking/research/current/tacfp/curriculum

Scales and other instruments

Cognitive assessment instruments

Rowland Universal Dementia Assessment Scale (RUDAS): http://www.dementia-assessment.com.au/cognitive/RUDAS_scale.pdf and http://www.dementia-assessment.com.au/cognitive/rudas_scoring.pdf

Standardised Mini-Mental State Examination (SMMSE): http://www.ihpa.gov.au/internet/ihpa/publishing.nsf/Content/smmse-lp

The General Practitioner assessment of COGnition (GPCOG): http://www.gpcog.com.au/

Depression screening

Geriatric Depression Scale: http://www.dementia-assessment.com.au/depression/
geriatric_depression_scale_short.pdf

Other scales from chapters in the book.

Index